EBURY PRESS

THE SKINCARE ANSWER BOOK

Dr Jaishree Sharad is an internationally renowned celebrity cosmetic dermatologist practising in Mumbai for twenty-three years. She is a TEDx speaker, and the founder and director of Skinfinitii Aesthetic Skin and Laser Clinic in Mumbai. Dr Jaishree is an international mentor for the mentorship programme of the American Society for Dermatologic Surgery. She has been the only Indian on the board of directors of the International Society of Dermatologic Surgery. She is the ex-vice president of the Cosmetic Dermatology Society of India. She is a highly sought-after international faculty for fillers, Botox, anti-aging treatments and Lasers. This is her third book.

'I have known Jaishree for over a decade and have seen her travel to various countries to give lectures at dermatology conferences and represent our country. It gives me immense pride to see a lady do this at such a young age. I am glad she has come out with her third book on common skin queries and am told it is a compilation of legitimate questions asked to her by her followers on social media. I wish her the very best. A book on skincare for all ages. In admiration and love'—Amitabh Bachchan

'Dr Jaishree Sharad is a celebrity dermatologist who does not require certification. Numerous well-known clients on her long list attest to her reliability. If only I were on the list now. I've known her for a while, and I really appreciate the singing ability she also possesses. May she achieve even more acclaim in the future'—Jaya Bachchan, actor and parliamentarian

'Jaishree is the best dermatologist I have known. I wish her all the best for her book. I am sure it will be handy for one and all. Love you, Jaishree. Go conquer'—Dimple Kapadia, actor

'People should know how to maintain their skin and hair. It is such an important thing for both women and men. I am sure this book will be brilliant. I'm so proud of you, Jaishree beta. She is so thorough and "*Main all the best bolti hoon aapki book ke liye*" and I'll be the first buyer and I will definitely read page to page. Love you, take care darling'—Mumtaz, actor

'At my age, when people complement me and say my skin is looking nice, I just want to say I want to bless Dr Jaishree Sharad, because I have always suffered from bad skin and acne throughout my life and it was only after I met her that my complete complexion changed. She has just done wonders without any Botox or fillers. I'm glowing, and it's only because of her and the radical, new, innovative treatments that she has used on my skin. I would say blindly follow her and whatever she says in the book because no one knows skin and hair better than her'—Farah Khan, director

'Dear Jaishree, congratulations for your new book. I bet it's gonna be great. All the best. I am dying to read it. You are one of the best skin doctors in the country. God bless you'—Sanjay Dutt, actor

'Your skin is the largest organ in your body and, honestly, a very important one. My skincare regime has evolved a lot over time—from an almost close to nothing regime to an extensive one to now keeping it super simple and to the bare minimum. Doc has been a one-point contact whenever my skin is under any kind of stress. As actors, our lifestyles are super unpredictable—shooting at odd hours, jumping time zones to shooing in the heart of pollution sometimes—all of this and more can contribute to a lot of stress and eventually cause the skin to respond with stress too. So whether it's on a lazy Sunday or in the middle of the night, I know Doc will always be there for me and my skin. And for that I am super grateful'—Alia Bhatt, actor

'Well, here's wishing Jaishree all the very best and congratulations for her third book. I'm sure this will be a bestseller! You truly have cracked the code of how to solve everyone's problems regarding skin and hair. Thank you for constantly looking after our skin and hair needs and, once again congratulations, my dear'—Malaika Arora, actor and fashion icon

'So, I remember meeting Jaishree for the first time and I had a wart. I must say what a great decision that was because after that, come what may, I never had a skin problem. Thank you so much, J, for always being there not just as my skin doctor who takes care of my skin but a dear friend. So, once again, thank you so much, Jaishree, for taking care of all of us the way you do especially as a skin doctor. Loads of love to you, you are just a rockstar'—Maniesh Paul, actor

'My dearest Jai! You are the best in your field but, to us you are family! Just a short note to thank you for making my face glow always. All the best for your third book. I'm sure it will come handy to one and all. Lots of love'—Riddhima Kapoor Sahni, fashion icon and jewellery designer

'Dr Jaishree is an absolute master at what she does. Her treatments always address the underlying issues curing from the root. If she's giving advice, I'm taking notes'—Shweta Bachchan Nanda, author, entrepreneur and fashion icon

'I've always been extremely particular about skincare, and over the past years I've gained so much more knowledge from Dr Jaishree. She's been someone who's always guided me through my skin journey. Someone I trust immensely and who never gets tired of answering my endless questions about skincare'—Athiya Shetty, actor

'Dr Jaishree is my safe place when it comes to my skin. I never believed in going to dermatologists until I met her and I never felt the need to go to any other because I got lucky the first time. I love the fact that she doesn't do unnecessary treatments. She keeps it simple yet super effective . . . the best doctor ever'—Sonal Chauhan, actor

'There's a lot I can say about Dr J. She's kind, passionate, dedicated to her work and inspiring. But what I love most about her is her work ethic. From experience, I can tell you that most dermatologists and cosmetologists think it's necessary to point out your "flaws" in order for them to suggest ways of "correcting" them, growing insecurities in you that never existed before. But Dr J is someone who has never once done that. Her approach to her practice is to make everyone feel worthy to begin with, addressing only the concerns we go to her with. No judgement whatsoever. She's been a boon at treating my acne when no one else could, and she is the first person I go to for skincare advice and is a constant source of inspiration. I cannot believe she's found time to write yet another book and share her knowledge with people who can't readily access her all the time. Dr J, congratulations! I have no idea if you even have time to sleep while doing all this, but I love that your smile and energy never fades'—Kalyani Priyadarshan, actor

'Dr Jaishree is a genius with a sharp eye and magical hands. Grateful to have her in my life'—Pragya Jaiswal, actor

'Dr Jaishree is not only our country's most formidable skincare expert and guide but is also a sensitive artist at her core, whose ability to find beauty in all forms pushes people to embrace their natural selves with kindness and holds them back from mindlessly chasing media-set cosmetic standards. Her no-fuss approach to beauty and wellness has had a huge impact on me. She gave me the kind of encouragement and healthy counsel most young people need. I am sure to always think of her as this rockstar–doctor with a gypsy soul! Love'—Sobhita Dhulipala, actor

'Jaishree is a superwoman. She is so good at what she does that I can trust her completely when it comes to any skin-related questions. Apart from being the best dermatologist, she's also one of my closest friends in Mumbai. She's smart, she's kind and she is brilliant at what she does. What else do you need? And I'm sure her book will be a superhit again just as she is *love*'—Priya Banerjee, actor

'Dr Jaishree is the best. She knows what's best for your type of skin and works around it accordingly'—Patralekha, actor

'Having a book on all the questions we have is absolutely amazing. Congrats, Dr Jaishree, on your third book and providing us with the much-needed information about our skin and hair! We all need help to maintain ourselves and now we all have you by our side. Love you'—Sunny Leone, actor

'For a stage artist like me, skincare is very important and for that I have Dr Jaishree, so I have nothing to fear. For the tiniest of skin problems, I just pick up the phone and call Dr Jaishree and she takes care of all my skin problems. She is a fantastic skin doctor and that is also the reason that her own skin keeps glowing all the time too'— Anup Jalota, musician and singer

'Dr Jaishree Sharad is absolutely the best and I'm following every instruction of hers regarding my skin. It's given me some great results: she makes your face and skin glow from within, and she knows exactly which treatment needs to be given to which skin type and is an absolutely wonderful human being besides being a great doctor'— Himesh Reshammiya, music composer and singer

'Jaishree is one of my closest friends. Apart from being absolutely brilliant at what she does, she heals people in more ways than one. Her warmth and compassion are her most beautiful qualities. I am certain that her thoughtful and expert insights in this book will answer many questions and open up many more minds towards a healthier and positive lifestyle'—Sheykhar Ravjiani, music composer and singer

'It's true when they say that the best thing you can wear is a good smile and good skin! The smile I have been blessed with the skin is thanks to Dr Jaishree. Radhika and I can't thank you enough for always serving us with happiness and treating all our (skin) problems'—Shaan, music composer and singer

'I have known Jaishree for almost two decades now and she is a close friend. Her deep knowledge of medicine, her progressive approach and, above all, her compassion makes her a truly special doctor. This new book will share her many insights into healthy skin, hair and healthy lifestyle'—Ehsaan Noorani, music composer and guitarist

'It has been years since I've looked no further than Dr Jaishree for my skin's well-being. Dr J's informed and holistic way of treatment has made me take care of my skin better. Her clinic has always been my go-to place when things have gone out of control with my skin'—Shalmali Kholgade, musician

'Trust is the biggest treasure anyone can give another . . . For most of the industry in particular, our face is our fortune, and there is no one I would trust more in this world then Dr Jaishree with my face and skin. I also trust that her next book will be just as magical as her last two and her! Love you always, xoxo'—Anusha Dandekar, singer and fashion icon

'I love taking care of myself, of my skin, my hair; it's important for my daily life, for my work, for my confidence and well-being. I need and want the best for myself, so when I need guidance, I call Dr Jaishree because I trust her experience, knowledge and her good heart. I'm happy that her new book of Q&A is coming out; it will make my life easier as I'll have the answers on my table. If you need that too . . . get her book, it's that easy! Enjoy yourself, enjoy your beauty'—Iulia Vantur, singer

'Dearest J, wish you the best for your third book. May you keep shining as bright as you make everyone's skin and hair shine. Lots of love'—Aditi Singh Sharma, singer

'Dear Jaishree, many congratulations to you on the new book. I'm really looking forward to reading it and getting all the insights on skin and hair care'—Priya Saraiya, singer and lyricist

'Dr Jaishree Sharad is an amazing combination of an excellent doctor and a great friend who loves and understands music as well. It's commendable the way she handles all her patients with a smile and confidence. According to me she is the best dermatologist. I wish her all the best, success and good health so she can make everyone feel good and look beautiful'—Pandit Rakesh Chaurasia, flautist

'Doc, congratulations on your third book. Can't wait to get my hands on it! Lots of love'—Ahan Shetty, actor

'Jaishree, also J for me, is a friend and a dermat later. I have to be honest, she's the most approachable, easy to speak doctor, and that is very important, especially in the field she is in. Everything to do with dermatology is elective, and it's important to have a doctor to guide you honestly. The first time I met her, she told me there was no need to do anything invasive, let's just holistically go slow and take care of my skin. And that's what I loved about her'—Karan Tacker, actor

'Skinfiniti has been home for years now. Dr Jaishree is my go-to person for all skin-related issues as I trust her completely. She never over-medicates and the little time we get together is always a bonus! Love you, Doc'—Aanya Singh, actor

'Dr Jaishree is absolutely extraordinary! Her level of knowledge, experience, professionalism and genuine concern are some of the characteristics that set her apart and make her the top doctor that she is! Every appointment is so well organized and smooth. She always understands what I'm looking to get done and gets me the results that I'm looking for each and every time. Even when I'm travelling and unable to visit her, I know I can always reach out to her for her recommendations on whom to see or what to do in the interim. Her genuine care for her patients' best interests at all times is definitely what makes her unique, as that in today's world is a rarity. I've been across the world and have yet to find someone of her calibre. There truly just aren't any words to explain how much gratitude I have for Dr Jaishree'—Jobanpreet Singh, actor

'Dr Jaishree Sharad has been of immense help every time I start a new project and in general for my usual skin appointments.

Highly appreciate her advice and already waiting to go back for my next appointment'—Gurfateh Pirzada, actor

'Here's wishing Dr Jaishree all the best for the new book that's coming out on skin and hair. It's apparently a question–answer book, so I'm sure all your questions can be answered. Who other than Dr Jaishree to answer those questions? I mean, she is the best, isn't it?'—Gaurav Chopra, actor

'What do I say about Dr Jaishree Sharad? To sum it up in 2–3 lines is impossible. To keep it simple and short, [she is] the best skin doctor in the whole world and this is not an exaggeration. I say this not only because she has a cure and remedy for everything, but also because she understands all skin types and recommends solutions accordingly, keeping all factors in mind, including one's pocket. Love and luck always'—Ayush Anand, actor

'Getting the right answers from the best doctor is what every patient requires and that's why Dr Sharad is the best doctor to go to! It has always been the best experience getting treatments done from Dr Sharad who makes it easy, comfortable and gentle. All the best with your new book, Doctor. You've scored a hattrick'—Geeta Basra, actor and model

'Skin is your most prominent indicator of general health. It's crucial to pay attention and take care of it, to take care of you. Dr Jaishree is my go-to guide for all things keeping my skin radiant and healthy'—Avantika Dassani, actor

'Can't do anything skin-related without getting Jaishree's opinion first. I never hesitate before approaching her with any concerns for me or my friends and family. No matter where in the world she is or how busy, J will always take out the time to be there for her clients. Everyone at her clinic does such a good job at keeping up with your treatments and ensuring you see the best results'—Alizeh Agnithotri, actor

'She's back with another one! As someone who's suffered with acne-prone skin for a while now, I have only Dr Jaishree to thank for helping me turn it around and get my confidence back. You truly are the best in the business! Thank you for sharing your knowledge with all of us. Lots of love'—Karan Kapadia, actor and rapper

'Over the years Jaishree has not only been one of the most amazing people with skincare for skin ailments for me and my family but also, in a world where everyone selling you 1000 different plans, I find Jaishree to be the most authentic, honest and incredibly knowledgeable in her field. As a friend, over the years I am yet to meet anybody who is constantly updating themselves and is constantly inquiring and researching to be the best that they could possibly be. So, in my life, out of the many people I have met, she is by far one of the best doctors I've come across in my life'—Cyrus Sahukar, actor

'My only solution for anyone around me when they talk of skin or hair care is Dr J. Her treatments and routines are so easy and have worked so well on me that nobody can question the incredible results'—Veer Pahariya, actor

'Dr Jaishree, many congratulations on the publishing of your third book. It's a remarkable feat for any woman and you, being a doctor and juggling so many roles at home and on the work front, it gives me great pride to know you personally and to be your patient. As a doctor, you are an approachable and kind specialist who has a lot of compassion for patients. As a woman, you inspire me because of all the wonderful things you have done and achieved for yourself, going from strength to strength. Loads of wishes'—Ishita Arun, actor

'A doc that's amazing! Big congratulations to you. I am always amazed, and this I'm genuinely saying that I'm always amazed by your capacity to put your knowledge and wisdom out there in the world for. I'm sure this third book of yours would be very helpful for people, and this would be something that we all should keep as our handbook on our coffee table or use it as our go-to book for any kind of concern or any kind of a quick answer to any of our concern, or just to flip through the pages of the book to draw something from the pool of amazing wisdom that you have. So, I wish you all the best, big congratulations and hats off to you. Keep this going, more power to you'—Priyansh Jora, actor

'Dr Jaishree Sharad is not a dermatologist, she's a dream-maker. She makes everyone's dreams come true. She makes everyone shine brighter'—Rohini Iyer, Bollywood publicist and entrepreneur

'I'm so happy to hear that Dr Jaishree is coming out with her third book. Her book is something I pick up, my family picks up and my friends also buy, because it is not just meant for anyone who's going for some hi-fi treatment. It's a very simple book always which, has home remedies, dos and don'ts, very good explanations and the things you should do, should not do to take care of your skin and hair. I would recommend these books to anyone those who wants to just take care of their skin and hair and what they have to do to take care of themselves. I'm really happy and can't wait to read this third book as well. All the best, Jaishree'—Rohit Khilnani, journalist

'Jaishree approaches skincare with a holistic approach and empathy. She addresses the root problem and gently guides you into nurturing and nourishing your skin. She's Dr Feel Good'—Jitesh Pillai, editor and journalist

'When it comes to my skin, I trust no one more than Dr Jaishree. In fact, she is possibly the only Indian doctor or only South Asian doctor, rather, who is invited around the world to conferences on cosmetology and skin to give talks. She has also written textbooks which are part of the syllabus in medical schools where they teach subjects, and that is a good indication of her expertise in this field. Of course, there are many cosmetologists in India today, it's a booming industry. When you really look at a person's achievements on an international scale, I doubt there's anybody in South Asia or rather India who can match Jaishree's'—Shunali Shroff, author

'I got my lip and chin fillers from Dr Jaishree very recently and the experience was absolutely amazing! It was such a smooth, painless experience, and she walked me through each step while it was in process, which really helped me learn about it as well. Not to mention her absolutely warm, loving vibe which made me feel instantly comfortable. Upwards and onwards, Doc'—Anam Chashmawala, blogger and influencer

'Dr Jaishree is a doll. She is one of the most fabulous dermatologists in Mumbai and a beautiful human being. Her warmth is always so welcoming. Whenever I'm in a dire state with my skin, as I suffer from hyperpigmentation, she's my go-to doc. I have read her earlier book, which offers a huge insight into beauty and skin; now, I'm looking forward to her new book, as the line of aesthetic beauty and health keeps evolving and so are our questions. And who better to answer all those queries. Doc, looking forward to this precious insight into beauty inside and out. Congratulations'—Prerna Goel, fashion icon and influencer

'There is no one other than Dr Jaishree whom I trust with my skin and face. She has transformed my skin and has been the only one to effectively tackle any skin-related issues I've ever had. She's my go-to for everything skin-related, the best there is'—Samiksha Pednekar, fashion icon and influencer

'It is a blessing to find a doctor whom I can trust blindly, but it's a tremendous gift to have that someone also be as kind and gentle as Dr Jaishree'—Carla Ruth Dennis, model and influencer

'My dear J is the best dermatologist and friend I've had. For all skin issues I consult her with my eyes closed. I trust her completely. She has great knowledge of the field she is in and is forever evolving. She works tirelessly and deserves all the success and adulation. God bless her with happiness and success'—Namrata Dutt Kumar, trustee, Nargis Dutt Foundation

'A relationship that started as doctor–patient and ended up being family . . . It just shows the empathy and personal care with which she treats one and all. I know that apart from being the go-to cosmetic dermatologist for most Bollywood actors and so many others, she is a great academician and one of the very few Indian doctors who have an astute international reputation and respect amongst the medical community around the world. An ideal woman of substance, a mentor, a teacher, an amazing friend and an inspiration, to say the least'—Dr Yuvrajsingh Jadeja, Infertility specialist

THE
SKINCARE
ANSWER BOOK

Answers to the Most Frequently
Asked Skincare Questions

DR JAISHREE SHARAD

EBURY
PRESS

An imprint of Penguin Random House

EBURY PRESS

USA | Canada | UK | Ireland | Australia
New Zealand | India | South Africa | China

Ebury Press is part of the Penguin Random House group of companies
whose addresses can be found at global.penguinrandomhouse.com

Published by Penguin Random House India Pvt. Ltd
4th Floor, Capital Tower 1, MG Road,
Gurugram 122 002, Haryana, India

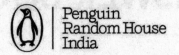

Penguin
Random House
India

First published in Ebury Press by Penguin Random House India 2023

Make-up for author by Bhavya Arora

ISBN 9780143461944

Typeset in Sabon LT Std by MAP Systems, Bengaluru, India
Printed at Replika Press Pvt. Ltd, India

www.penguin.co.in

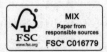

MIX
Paper from
responsible sources
FSC® C016779

Contents

Preface

To my parents . . . my constant guiding stars from heaven . . .

The world came to a standstill in March 2020 with COVID-19. From wishing for more than twenty-four hours in a day, suddenly twenty-four hours seemed like twenty-four years. In spite of cleaning the house, cooking, dishwashing, reading, completing my journal work as associate editor of a peer-reviewed cosmetic dermatology journal and even watching a movie on Netflix almost every day, I found myself sitting idle. And then I discovered a new hobby called 'scrolling Instagram'. I was amazed at the amount of information on skincare that was being churned every day—a lot of it confusing and inauthentic, and some could even be detrimental for the largest organ of our body aka the skin. I also saw the growing interest in skincare amongst people. However, the amount of knowledge which was being suddenly put out there could be confusing or even overwhelming for the reader. Youngsters who consulted me online during the COVID lockdown had bought innumerable products that caused more harm to their skin than good. Watching others' reels and posts created FOMO (fear of missing out), which led them to overrule their logic and buy into inauthentic advice. I realised there may be thousands of people influenced by social media, using wrong products or opting for unnecessary skincare, spending their time, energy and money at the cost of their precious skin. I found it very disturbing. Dermatologists get their degree after completing MBBS, followed by two to three years of post-graduation. It doesn't end there because science is evolving. To keep up with it, we study and upgrade our scientific, research and evidence-based knowledge every day. We understand the anatomy, physiology and pathology of skin. We understand the connection of the skin with the internal organs. And, I think in the present era, where there are a plethora of beauty bloggers and influencers, there is no harm if a dermatologist resorts to social media to talk about the real deal on skin. In fact, it is our duty to help people distinguish the right from wrong when it comes to skincare. That's when I decided to use my free time to create content for social media—to be able to cultivate authentic, scientific awareness about skin and skincare amongst people. I started conducting Instagram live sessions and 'ask me' stories where I got the opportunity to interact with hundreds of people who reached out with their skin queries. This became a daily routine for me. In October 2020, my editor

Gurveen reached out to me with the idea of my third book on skin-related questions and answers. By then, I was writing a few chapters on fillers and Botox for two medical textbooks. So, I mulled over the idea over some time. Days passed, the lockdown ended and I got busier with clinics. Gurveen never stopped prodding and reminding me to take up the project. One fine evening, after almost a year, I was cleaning up my phone gallery when I came across the innumerable questions that my Instagram followers asked me in response to my stories. I realised I could use these for my book and that's when I wrote back to Gurveen in the affirmative. Over the next two months, I compiled all the legitimate questions on skincare asked by my social media followers. I started writing elaborate answers to these questions one by one and, before I realized, my question-answer book on skincare was ready, majorly with the help of my Instagram handle @drjaishreesharad.

Chapter 1 is all about getting to know the basics of skin. If you get stuck at your favorite beauty store, trying to pick the right product for your skin type, then Chapter 2 is for you. It tells you how to identify your skin type. Is it okay to use a soap or is a face wash mandatory to wash your face? Should you exfoliate your face at all? Is a moisturizer necessary in the hot summers? Is a sunscreen important when you are indoors? If these questions confuse you, then Chapters 3, 4, 5 and 6 will unveil all your queries on cleansers, exfoliation, moisturizers, and sunscreens, respectively. Chapter 7 is something everybody suddenly seems to know. Yes, 'Actives', as they are known on social media, are active ingredients present in skincare products. They have been existing for decades and dermatologists have routinely prescribed them in their skincare prescriptions depending on the patient's requirements. Thanks to the digital world and social media as well as the innumerable cosmetics companies emerging and marketing extensively, actives have become a household name now. Active ingredients may be available in formulations of serums, creams, lotions and even cleansers. The efficacy of active formulations depends on the concentration of the active ingredient, its bio-availability (penetration rate for an active to reach its site of action) and the research that has gone behind it. The truth and myths about active ingredients lie in this chapter. This is followed by yet another talked about topic, 'serums', which is an extension of Chapter 7. Serum first or moisturizer first? Chapter 9 will teach you how to layer your products on your skin the right way to get the maximum out of the product you apply. Have you seen some people with fabulous faces, but their neck or hands and feet are wrinkled and old? Chapters 10 and 11 are about the often neglected neck, hands and feet. Nail art is in vogue these days but if you do not take care of your nails, this art is of no use. Chapter 12 is about nail care. Hair symbolizes health and personality and is the crown one never wants to take off. Chapter 14 has answers to all your questions on hair fall while Chapter 13 is all about hair removal methods. Chapter 15 is a must read for all genders and all age groups because this menace starts in your teens and continues till menopause. And you got it right, it's acne, the most psychologically traumatizing skin issue faced by most people. Chapters 16 and 17 are all about rectifying your skin to go make-up free. Here, I answer all questions on skin texture and hyperpigmentation, from acne scars to pores, to dark circles, dark lips, dark elbows, dark neck and everything in between. Do you want to wake up every morning and smile at yourself, feel confident and look youthful? Then you must read Chapter 18. It reveals all about aging skin, fine lines, wrinkles, sagging and the right age for treatments and how to choose the right treatment for yourself. From gua sha to dermarollers, Chapter 19 will tell you if these home gadgets sculpt your faces or are they a marketing gimmick. Did you know that your skin type may change with a change in season? Well, if you didn't, Chapter 20 is for you. Some of the most common skin conditions like eczemas and fungal infections are discussed in Chapter 21. And Chapter 22 winds up with all the common queries I get asked by most people.

Happy reading! With love,
Dr J aka Jaishree Sharad

1

Basics of Skin

'Your skin is the blueprint of your internal organs. Keep it healthy and safe.'

—Jaishree Sharad

To understand my answers to your questions, it is important to understand the skin a little better.

Our skin is made up of the upper epidermis and the lower dermis. The epidermis comprises layers of cells; the upper layers form the stratum corneum, which is made up of dead cells, lipids, the protein keratin, urea, salts and 30 per cent water. Lipids are oily, waxy or fatty compounds that are insoluble in water. The dead skin cells are laid like bricks, and there are lipids between the bricks which act like mortar. This brick-and-mortar arrangement forms a protective barrier in the skin. The major lipids that form the multilamellar barrier of

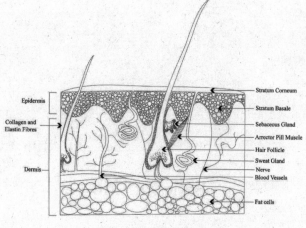

The skin diagram

the skin consist of 50 per cent ceramides, 25 per cent cholesterol and 15 per cent fatty acids (FAs). The skin also contains NMFs (natural moisturizing factors) made up primarily of amino acids, electrolytes and minerals.

Beneath the epidermis lies the dermis. The dermis contains the oil or sebaceous glands and sweat glands. It also has the collagen and elastin fibres, which form the basic framework of the skin and support the skin structure. Collagen fibres are made up of protein and are responsible for the skin's firmness. Elastin fibres keep the skin tight. The dermis also contains an important molecule called hyaluronic acid—a polysaccharide glycosaminoglycan—that builds moisture in the skin. It has the unique capacity to bind and retain water molecules.

Apart from covering the body, the skin performs an important function—it forms a physical barrier that protects the internal organs from the environment. It also protects the body from ultraviolet (UV) rays, mechanical damage, microorganisms and pollution. It regulates temperature and is a sensory organ that helps perceive pain, touch, pressure, vibration, heat and cold. It is an endocrine organ. Endocrine organs make and release hormones that travel in the bloodstream and control the actions of other cells or organs. Growth hormone, insulin-like growth factor-1, neuropeptides, sexual steroids, glucocorticoids and vitamin D are some hormones that are active in the skin.

The skin also helps in the excretion of water, urea and ammonia through sweat. The skin secretes products such as sebum. The skin has an immune system that protects the body from toxins, infections and even cancer.

Now let us look at skin colour. Skin colour is determined by two types of pigments, that is, melanin, called Eumelanin and Phaeomelanin. Eumelanin is the brown-black pigment in the skin cells while phaeomelanin is the yellow-red pigment. The relative ratio of eumelanin (brown-black) to pheomelanin (yellow-red) as well as the number of melanosomes within melanocytes determine skin colour. Melanocytes are cells in the skin that produce the pigment called melanin. Melanosomes are organelles which contain melanin within the melanocytes. Darker skin types have a higher quantity of eumelanin whereas fairer skin types have more phaeomelanin. The overall melanin density correlates with the darkness of skin, and it increases with sun exposure. Populations living closer to the equator tend to develop a greater proportion of eumelanin, while populations living further from the equator are relatively richer in pheomelanin. Eumelanin is a UV-absorbent, antioxidant and free radical scavenger. Conversely, phaeomelanin produces free radicals in response to UV radiation, accelerating carcinogenesis. Hence dark skin is more of a blessing.

Our skin is a window to our inner health.

A whole lot of disorders of the internal organs manifest signs and symptoms on the skin. For example, if one has diabetes, one is more prone to infections and may also develop a condition called acanthosis nigricans (described in detail in the chapter on skin tone) in the skin folds. If you have hypothyroidism, you may experience dry skin, hair fall and even hyperpigmentation. If you have polycystic ovary syndrome (PCOS), you may be prone to acne, hair fall and hirsutism. Yellow discoloration of skin can be a sign of jaundice. Hence it is important to listen to your skin. If you see anything subnormal, it is a good idea to consult a dermatologist.

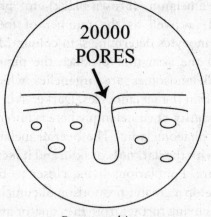

Pores on skin

FUN FACTS ABOUT YOUR SKIN

The skin is the largest and heaviest organ of the body. It covers approximately 20 square feet of surface area.

An average square inch of skin contains twenty blood vessels, 650–700 sweat glands and more than 1,000 nerve endings.

The skin makes up around one-seventh of a person's body weight.

The face itself has approximately 20,000 pores. Pores are the openings of the oil glands.

A person sheds around 500 million skin cells each day.

2

Skin Types

'Loving your skin isn't vanity, it's sanity.'
—André Gide

One's skin type is determined by the number of sebaceous glands, the climate and hormonal changes that occur in the body. Skin can be oily, dry, combination, sensitive or normal. The right skincare routine for an individual depends on their skin type. With the plethora of skincare products available in the market, it could get very confusing for a person to decide which products would suit them. Hence it is important to understand one's skin type.

1. Is there a test to identify one's skin type?

Wash your face in the morning as soon as you wake up and do not apply anything for the next hour. If your skin feels dry to the touch after an hour or if it is flaky, you have dry skin. If you blot your face with a tissue paper and it gets smudged with oil, you have oily skin. If the tissue paper is transparent only in patches, you have combination skin. If your skin breaks out into an itchy rash very easily, you have sensitive skin. If you develop acne, blackheads or whiteheads easily, especially upon applying a new product, you have acne-prone skin. If you develop dark marks on your skin easily after any cuts, wounds or acne, etc., you have pigment-prone skin. If none of the above happen, you have normal skin.

2. My skin is dry in the morning but becomes oily after two to three hours. What is my skin type?

This means you have oily skin. When you wash your face in the morning, it takes some time for the sebum from the sebaceous gland to reach the skin surface. Through the day you will find your skin to be shiny and even greasy on a hot day.

3. I have acne only on some parts of my face. I don't know whether my skin is oily or normal or dry. How do I buy products for my skin?

You probably have combination skin, which means that you have oil glands concentrated in some parts of your face, making those parts oily and other parts normal. There are hybrid products that can be used on combination

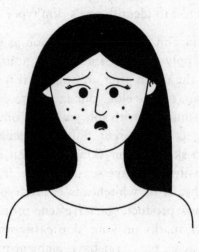

Oily skin

skin. You can even use oil-free, non-comedogenic products which are meant for normal skin.

4. My skin feels dry but I get pimples very often. What is my skin type?

You have dry, acne-prone skin. This means you break out into acne with the application of products, a change in the climate or a change in hormone levels. You should buy neutral products that are not too creamy or oily so that your skin remains moisturized without getting clogged and breaking out into acne. Use a gentle, foam-free face wash that does not strip the moisture from your skin. Do not skip using a moisturizer. However, use a light moisturizer or gel-based moisturizer both during the day and at night. You should avoid moisturizers that contain occlusives

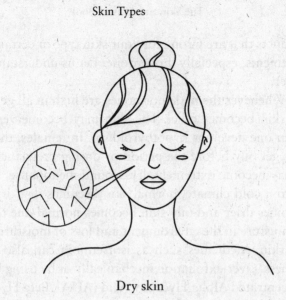

Dry skin

such as oil, petrolatum, waxes and lanolin, which can clog your pores easily. Look for products with labels such as non-comedogenic, water-based or oil-free. At the same time, do not use products with salicylic acid because they can increase the dryness on your face. You can opt for alpha hydroxy acids such as lactic acid and mandelic acid or polyhydroxy acids instead. These cause gentle chemo exfoliation but will also keep your skin moisturized.

5. My skin is normal, but whenever I go to a cold climate my skin becomes very dry and my lips chap. So, do I have dry skin or combination skin?

While your basic skin type is always determined by your genes, it can alter with a change in hormones or climate, certain medicines, over-exfoliation, the use of products that are wrong for your skin type or certain skin treatments, especially if overdone. Let us understand this better.

Whenever the male hormones are high in all genders, the skin becomes oilier. The skin may become very dry when one develops hypothyroidism. In females, the skin may get oily before the period or during pregnancy, and it may become extremely dry around menopause. If you go to a cold climate, normal skin becomes dry, dry skin becomes drier and oily skin becomes normal due to lack of moisture in the environment and loss of moisture from the skin. Medicines such as isotretinoin can also cause dryness. Over-exfoliation mechanically or by using highly concentrated Alpha Hydroxy Acid (AHA), Beta Hydroxy Acid (BHA) or retinol, or by opting for chemical peels or Laser treatments very frequently (like every week to ten days) can also dry out your skin.

6. I have noticed that my skin feels normal and lovely after my period, but about ten days before my period, it starts to become oily again. Can skin type change like this?

Yes, your skin may change depending on the phase of your menstrual cycle. Right after your period, your skin is at its best. It is neither dry nor oily. This is because there is a dip in the progesterone hormone and a rise in oestrogen in the follicular phase of your menstrual cycle. The follicular phase is followed by the ovulatory phase. This is when both oestrogen and progesterone are high. The next phase is the luteal phase, which occurs ten to twelve days before your period, when the oestrogen dips and the progesterone rises, making the skin oilier and prone to acne.

7. Are dry skin and dehydrated skin the same?

Absolutely not! Dry skin is genetically predetermined and depends on the number of oil glands in your skin. So, when the skin is dry, there is a lack of oil or sebum in your skin. Dehydrated skin, on the other hand, lacks water. The skin gets its water from its deeper layers as well as the environment. So, if you do not drink enough water, the skin tries to take its water from the environment. If there is less moisture or humidity and the climate is dry, the skin is unable to absorb moisture from the air too, thereby becoming dehydrated. Skin can also become dehydrated if the skin barrier is compromised due to extremely dry weather, pollution, incorrect use of products, overzealous exfoliation, etc. This results in loss of water from the skin. The inability of the stratum corneum to absorb water from the atmosphere also results in dehydrated skin.

8. I have very dry skin on my body but my face always seems oily. Is this possible?

Yes, your face can be oily while your body is dry. Oiliness depends on the number and distribution of sebaceous glands on the face and body. So, if your face has a greater number of oil glands that are constantly secreting sebum, your face will be oily. On the contrary, the concentration of sebaceous glands on your body may be proportionately less, which is why the skin on your body is dry.

9. Whenever I apply a new product on my face, I get pimples. What do I do for my sensitive skin?

Sensitive skin will break out into an itchy red rash with the application of a new product. Since you develop acne upon applying any new product, you have acne-prone skin. Check the labels on the products before you buy them. Your product should be non-comedogenic, oil-free, water-based and should not contain occlusive ingredients such as oils, petrolatum, lanolin and wax.

10. I had very oily skin when I was young. I have just turned forty-five, and now my skin feels flaky and dry. Why is that so?

As we get older, the hormones in our body change. Closer to reaching menopause, oestrogen dips. This results in less oil production by the sebaceous glands. The skin's ability to retain water, regenerate collagen and maintain the skin cell cycle of twenty-eight days slows down. Therefore it is possible for your skin to be oily when you are young and then naturally become drier as you grow older.

11. I tend to get itching and rashes on my face randomly. Is it because I have dry skin?

You probably have sensitive skin. Sensitive skin can get red, itchy, bumpy or flaky with a change in climate, skincare products, cosmetics, perfumes, contact with rubber, leather, metal, pollen, dust or pollution. Always use soap-free face and body washes. Avoid hot water, steam, sauna, bubble baths and scrubs, all of which can dehydrate or dry your skin, making it more sensitive. Moisturize your skin adequately. Stay away from alcohol-based products. If you have sensitive skin, allergies to parabens and fragrance are very common. So, opt for fragrance-free and paraben-free cosmetics and skincare products. Always check with the dermatologist before you start using any new skincare products.

12. Whenever I get acne or an injury, even if I don't touch it, it leaves dark spots behind. Is my skin type sensitive?

No, you do not have sensitive skin. Your skin is prone to hyperpigmentation. Usually, darker skin is more prone to pigmentation because it has more phaeomelanin, the pigment responsible for skin colour. Baumann's skin-type classification labels this skin as pigmented skin type. Melanocytes (pigment-forming cells in the skin) produce more melanin upon sun exposure, injury to the skin or any skin abuse. So, when you get acne, injuries, cuts, scratches, boils or any skin lesions, they heal with dark spots. You must always be gentle with your skin. Never over-exfoliate and use a broad-spectrum sunscreen in the right quantity every single day. Take supplements of vitamin C and antioxidants as well. Pigment-lightening creams, chemical peels and the Q-switched Nd:YAG Laser are treatment options for resistant blemishes and dark spots.

RAPID FIRE

1. My skin feels dry when I go to a cold climate. It feels slightly oily when I am in Mumbai where humidity is high. What's my skin type?

You probably have an oily T-zone which is why your skin feels slightly oily in humid weather but gets dry in cold weather.

2. I get acne the moment I apply most creams or make-up on my skin. Is my skin sensitive?

You have acne-prone skin. Sensitive skin breaks out into an itchy or red rash, not acne.

3. I get acne very often. I have read that those with acne have oily skin, but my skin feels dry. What's my skin type?

You can have dry skin and acne due to a hormonal imbalance such as PCOS or insulin resistance.

4. Do people with oily skin age slower?

Not at all. Aging depends on genes, hormones, climate, pollution, food, stress, sleep, exercise, medicines, smoking, lifestyle but not on your skin type.

5. Which is the best skin type?

A normal or balanced skin type which is neither too oily nor too dry is the best.

3

Cleansers

'If you don't take care of this the most magnificent machine that you will ever be given . . . where are you going to live?'

—Karyn Calabrese

The idea of cleansing dates back to the origin of human race, only the ritual was perhaps different. In ancient times, people used bone, stone and plant extracts to scrape the skin. Soaps were made as early as in 2000 BC and can be found in Sumerian clay tablets. Phoenicians used animal fat and tree ash to make soap in 600 BC. The Greek physician Galen (130–200 AD) and the eighth-century chemist Gabiribne Hayyan were the first to have written about the use of soap as a body-cleansing agent.

The importance of cleansing our skin to maintain skin hygiene needs to be understood and practised.

1. What is a face wash and how often should I use one?

A face wash is a cleanser which helps remove water soluble substances such as sweat salts, microorganisms, dead cells as well as water-insoluble substances such as sebum, dirt, grime, environmental impurities and oil-based make-up from the skin surface. Cleansers contain ingredients which are capable of emulsifying water insoluble substances into finer particles and making these fat-soluble impurities water soluble. Ideally, you should cleanse your face twice a day—once in the morning and once at night—using a face wash keeping in mind your existing skin conditions—such as acne or rosacea—and the climate that you live in.

2. What type of face wash should I use for dry skin?

If you have dry, flaky skin, opt for a gentle face wash with added moisturizers and super fatty acids including petrolatum, lanolin, mineral oil, cocoa butter, glycerin, shea butter and ceramides. You can also use products that contain natural ingredients such as jojoba oil, coconut oil, aloe vera, soybean oil and olive oil. Avoid using soaps with a high pH value, antibacterial or exfoliating properties as they have the potential to irritate the skin.

3. What type of face wash should I use for oily skin?

Those with oily, acne-prone skin should opt for a face wash that foams mildly. Select a face wash with exfoliating ingredients such as salicylic acid, glycolic acid and lactic acid, or botanicals including aloe vera, tea tree oil or grape seed oil, as they can help balance excessive oil production. However, if you are using anti-acne creams or are consuming acne-specific medication, opt for a gentle, non-soap cleanser for your skin.

4. What type of face wash should I use for combination skin?

If you have a combination skin type—such as an oily T-zone with dry skin—pick a face wash that is neither too drying nor too moisturizing. Alternatively, use a specific kind of cleanser ideal for your oily T-zone, and a moisturizing one for the rest of your face.

5. What type of face wash should I use for sensitive skin?

Do you tend to develop a rash after using a face wash you buy off the shelf? If yes, you have sensitive skin. I would advise that you stay away from medicated face washes, along with those containing fragrance or alcohol, as these ingredients often irritate the skin. Instead, pick a face wash with neutral to acidic pH, which has moisturizing properties. Micellar water works best for sensitive skin. It absorbs dust and impurities, thus cleansing the skin thoroughly.

6. Should we use cold water or lukewarm water to wash the face?

When you pour hot water on the skin, the water evaporates and takes away the moisture from the skin, thus leaving the skin dehydrated. Cold water, on the

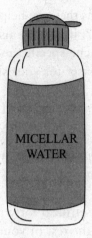

other hand, won't dissolve and remove embedded dirt and grime. Hence it is advisable to use normal water or mildly lukewarm water to wash the face.

7. How many times should I wash my face with a face wash during the summer?

You can use a face wash up to three times a day in summer if you have normal, combination or oily skin. If you have

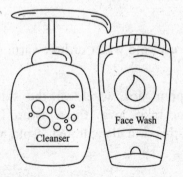

sensitive skin, wash your face one to two times a day with a soap-free cleanser. If you have dry skin, you can wash your face twice a day.

8. Is it necessary to use toner for acne-prone skin? And what does it do to our skin?

A toner is not an essential skincare step if you cleanse your face well with a face wash meant for acne-prone skin. However, if you want to use a toner because you have very oily skin, you may do so. A toner is known to double cleanse, reduce the oils and unclog the pores.

9. Is oil cleansing good for oily skin? If yes, which oils can one use?

If you have oily skin, you must avoid oil-based cleansers. So, definitely do not opt for oil cleansing. You may end up clogging your pores, resulting in acne or milia or

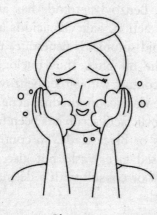

Cleansing

sometimes even folliculitis, which is an infection of the hair follicle.

10. Can a brightening face wash help reduce the dark patches on the skin?

Skin-brightening face washes containing vitamin C, curcumin, niacinamide, white daffodils or kojic acid may help in cleansing the face and have an immediate brightening effect. However, having these ingredients in a face wash does not reduce hyperpigmentation. One reason for this is that a face wash is in contact with the skin for a short time only, and a second reason is that the concentration of the active ingredient in the face wash is very low.

11. I use a salicylic acid-based face wash, but my acne keeps coming back. What cleanser should I use?

Cleansers containing 2 per cent salicylic acid or 5 per cent benzoyl peroxide are prescribed for people with acne or acne-prone skin. Benzoyl peroxide has an antibacterial and comedolytic action. Salicylic acid is a beta hydroxy acid, which is lipid-soluble. It penetrates the hair follicle and dislodges the oil plug, thus unclogging the pore. However, short contact with either benzoyl peroxide or a salicylic acid face wash cannot reduce acne or whiteheads. A 2 per cent salicylic acid scrub has been found to reduce open comedones or blackheads. So continue to use the salicylic acid-based face wash, but also use a salicylic acid-based serum or consult with a dermatologist to get your acne treated.

12. Can I use besan to wash my face instead of a face wash?

If you have oily or normal skin you can use besan (chickpea flour) to cleanse your face. Besan has mild exfoliating properties. It can also reduce the oiliness of your skin. However, it can cause dryness of the skin. Hence it is not good for dry skin or sensitive skin. Using besan every day on acne-prone skin will also aggravate the acne. Last but not the least, there are no scientific studies on the usage of besan as a cleanser.

13. What should the ideal pH of a cleanser be?

The normal pH value of skin on most of our face and body lies between 4.7 and 5.75. So the ideal pH of a cleanser should be between 4.5 and 6. This acidic-to-neutral pH helps preserve the normal flora of the skin as well as retains moisture yet cleanses the skin thoroughly. However, most cleansers do not mention their pH value. Generally, foam-based cleansers have a higher pH, and they can make the skin alkaline and dry. Soap-free cleansers usually have an acidic or low pH and are safer for dry and sensitive skin.

14. Can we use micellar water instead of a cleanser?

Micellar water is a water-based cleanser with a mild surfactant or cleansing agent.

A micelle is a minute structure with a hydrophobic and hydrophilic end, dissolved in a water solution. Particles or substances with a special affinity for water are known as hydrophilic. Substances or particles that naturally repel water are known as hydrophobic. It helps clean the dirt, grime and debris from the skin without altering the skin's pH. Micellar water can be used to remove make-up as well. It can also be used as a perfect cleanser for aging or sensitive skin.

15. How does one choose a good cleanser for aging skin?

As we age, the skin tends to get drier because it loses its ability to retain moisture, and the lipids in the skin tend to reduce. So, you have to opt for a cleanser that is gentle, does not foam too much and does not contain alcohol or fragrance or any abrasive or irritant ingredient. Opt for a soap-free cleanser that removes the dirt, excess oil, debris and make-up without drying the skin. Opting for a cleanser that makes the skin squeaky clean is not the right choice. No matter what an advertiser promises, a skin cleanser will not prevent or reverse signs of aging.

16. Is double cleansing necessary?

Double cleansing is a method by which two different types of cleansers are used to wash the face. A cleansing oil or balm is used to remove the oils and make-up as well as sunscreen and pave way for the regular cleanser to remove the rest of the dirt, grime, sweat salts, etc. Now, double cleansing is not really necessary if you use a good cleanser that can remove all the oil, dirt, grime, make-up and sweat salts from your face. You can even use the same cleanser twice or use a washcloth or a brush to deep cleanse. Double cleansing may be done if there is thick, oil-based make-up on the face or a mineral sunscreen that does not come off easily with a normal cleanser or if one has been exposed to a lot of pollution and dust for long hours. In such situations, a cleansing oil or cleansing balm is first used to remove the make-up or the oily ingredient on the face. The cleansing oil or cleansing balm usually contains an emulsifier, which allows the oil to mix with water and form a milky emulsion. This helps rinse the cleanser from the skin easily without leaving a greasy residue. This is followed by the use of a regular cleanser.

17. What is a cleansing oil?

Cleansing oils are used to remove heavy make-up, excess oil and thick debris on the skin. They contain a mild surfactant, but the main stars are the oils. Oils work as solvents (a group of ingredients that can dissolve similar substances) and dissolve the sebum as well as oily make-up, thus helping to deep-cleanse the face. Avoid fragrance-based cleansing oils especially if you have sensitive skin. If you have acne or acne-prone skin or oily skin, you should use the oil only to remove eye make-up and use a regular cleanser for the rest of the face.

18. Since I have acne-prone oily skin, is it okay to wash my face five to six times a day?

Washing one's face frequently will not reduce the oiliness and acne. In fact, the skin will get more irritated and inflamed. The sebaceous glands will secrete more oil as a defence mechanism. Hence it is better to wash your face only twice a day.

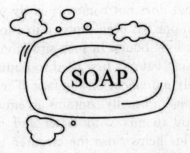

19. I have been asked to use a soap-free cleanser but my face does not feel clean after I wash it. Should I continue with the cleanser?

Cleansers that produce a lot of foam and lather can make the pH of the skin more alkaline and thus dry the skin. They are no more effective than soap-free or non-foamy cleansers. Also, sometimes the ingredients used to produce lather can cause skin irritation and eczema. Soap-free cleansers clean just as well although you don't get the feeling of having cleaned the skin properly. So, if you have been asked to use a soap-free cleanser by a dermatologist, then you must follow his/her instructions.

20. Are soaps better than face washes or shower gels?

Soaps are derived from fatty acids and triglycerides (fats and oils). There are routine soaps that may increase the pH of the skin and make it alkaline and dry. Deodorant or antimicrobial bars have an added antibacterial agent to combat bacteria. These soaps have a pH between 9 and 10 and may cause skin irritation. They should be used only if prescribed by a physician, albeit for a short duration. Moisturizing soaps contain moisturizing agents such as lanolin or glycerine. Their pH is between 5 and 7, so they are non-irritant. They can be used if you have dry skin. However, if you really want to use a bar, use a syndet bar, which looks like a soap and cleanses even better without making the skin dry.

RAPID FIRE

1. I wash my face only with water. I have never used a face wash or soap. Is it okay?

Sebum, sweat salts, make-up, dirt, grime and environmental impurities may not be water-soluble. Hence cleansing with water alone is not enough. Please use a cleanser at least once a day.

2. Which is the best facewash?

There is no best one. What is good for you may not suit another person. However, opt for facewashes which do not contain fragrance, synthetic colours, alcohol or grainy exfoliators.

3. Can I use multani mitti to cleanse my face as it is too oily?

While it is alright to use multani mitti (Fuller's earth) once in a week if you have oily skin, using it daily will strip your natural oils and make your skin dry or sensitive.

4. I tend to sweat a lot. Do I have to use a face wash every time I sweat too much?

Not at all. Just splash your face with water or spray some thermal water mist to wash away the sweat salts.

5. I stay indoors the entire day. Do I still need to wash my face before sleeping?

You must use a cleanser or a facewash at least at bedtime. Sebum, sweat salts, dirt and dead cells accumulate on your skin throughout the day and need to be removed.

4

Exfoliation

> 'We are born with a clean soul. We need to exfoliate
> the layers of ego, anger and negativity from time to
> time to see the clean soul within just as we need to
> exfoliate our dead skin cells to see the radiant skin
> beneath.'
>
> —Jaishree Sharad

The process of exfoliation was probably first described
by the ancient Egyptians. They used pumice stone and
followed the dry body brushing technique to exfoliate
the skin mechanically. They also discovered chemical
exfoliants in the form of lactic acid derived from sour
milk and wine.

Ayurvedic medicine from India dates back to 5000
years and Gharsana or dry body brushing was introduced
in Ayurveda. Linen gloves and raw silk were also used to

mechanically scrub the skin. Coconut fibre is still used in various parts of India as a mechanical scrub.

Dried fibres of a gourd called silk squash were used by the traditional Chinese since ancient times. Ancient Greeks and Romans exfoliated using an instrument with a curved blade called a strigil, to remove dirt, sweat and oil before they bathed. The Turks used fire to singe the skin in an attempt to induce light exfoliation. American Indians used dried corn cobs, and Polynesian people would use crushed seashells.

Today, the market is flooded with physical as well as chemical exfoliants. While it is believed that exfoliation improves the appearance of skin, if not done right, it can actually harm the skin. The process of exfoliation should be gentle, adequate and done at regular intervals for better looking skin.

1. What is exfoliation and why is it necessary for the skin?

The skin has a natural cycle whereby the deeper layers of the epidermis reach the surface in twenty-eight days. When one is young, this natural process helps in shedding the dead skin and keeping the skin supple and radiant. With age, a bad lifestyle or excessive sun exposure, the skin loses its ability to follow this twenty-eight-day cycle and there is a build-up of dead skin on the surface, leading to a dull and dehydrated appearance of the skin and a rough texture. Sometimes the build-up of dead cells can clog the pores, leading to whiteheads and blackheads. In such conditions, it is important to exfoliate the skin. Exfoliation is a process by which the dead cells are removed from the outer layers of the skin.

2. What is the right way to exfoliate the face, feet and back?

Apply the exfoliating scrub on wet skin and, using your fingertips, massage it gently on the skin using small, circular motions. Do this for thirty seconds and rinse with normal or lukewarm water. Avoid hot water. Do not overdo the process as it may leave the skin irritated and red.

3. What are the methods of exfoliation?

Exfoliants remove the dead cells, sebum, dirt and grime, and help optimize the twenty-eight-day cell turnover cycle. This results in clear, smoother and brighter skin and an improvement in skin texture. There are three types of exfoliants, namely, physical, chemical and enzymatic.

Physical exfoliants are products containing small particles such as finely crushed nuts or fruit shells, powdered fruit rind or any sort of textured material such as a washcloth or a facial cleansing brush.

Dermaplaning

Chemical exfoliants are either AHAs such as glycolic acid, lactic acid or mandelic acid or BHAs such as salicylic acid.

AHAs are derived from natural substances and cause exfoliation. They remove the 'glue' that holds dead skin cells together, causing microexfoliation.

Glycolic acid is derived from sugarcane and is available in concentration of 5 to 10 per cent; it is safe for normal and oily skin. Those with dry skin can use lactic acid available in a concentration of 10 to 20 per cent. Lactic acid, also derived from milk, is moisturizing apart from being a mild chemical exfoliant.

Mandelic acid, which is derived from bitter almonds, has a larger molecule size than glycolic acid and penetrates the skin very slowly as compared to glycolic acid. Therefore it causes less irritation to the skin. A 10 per cent solution of mandelic acid can be safely used on normal, oily or combination skin.

Salicylic acid, a beta hydroxy acid, is lipid-soluble, which is great for oily and acne-prone skin because it unclogs the pores. It also has anti-inflammatory and antibacterial properties. A 2 per cent concentration of salicylic acid is safe to use at home.

The third type of exfoliants are enzymatic exfoliants. These are typically fruit enzymes such as papain (found in papaya) and bromelain (found in pineapple). They help in the process of exfoliation without causing irritation. Hence they can be used for those with sensitive skin. People with sensitive skin can also use a polyhydroxy acid, a milder combination of acids which don't cause irritation.

4. How many times should one exfoliate the skin?

If you have oily or acne-prone skin you can exfoliate twice a week, provided you are not taking any anti-acne tablets or using anti-acne creams. If you have blemishes and pigmentation, you can exfoliate about once in two weeks. Do not exfoliate more than that because excessive exfoliation can cause pigmentation. If you have dull, dry skin, you will damage the lipid barrier, which is the protective layer of the skin, and that will cause more sensitivity. Hence it is best to exfoliate once in a fortnight using the milder acids like lactic acid or polyhydroxy acid.

5. What are the tools and procedures for exfoliation?

Dermaplaning is one of the ways in which you can exfoliate your skin. A tiny scalpel is used to scrape off one layer of dead skin. This process removes facial hair and exfoliates the skin. Microdermabrasion is another way to exfoliate. It can be done on any skin area in need of exfoliation such as the face, neck, the back of the hands, legs and chest. It removes dead cells, resulting in smooth and radiant skin. Aluminum oxide crystals are used to exfoliate the skin. Chemical peels, which involve the application of a solution to the skin in a controlled manner to produce controlled exfoliation, can also be used. The solution may be an acid, a fruit extract, a botanical extract or even a milk extract. A chemical peel can be done on any part of the body but should only be done at skin clinics under a dermatologist's supervision. Face and body scrubs may also be used, which are usually applied at salons, but you can use DIY scrubs at home too using fruit extracts and oatmeal. Other tools such as silicon loofahs, Clarisonic brushes and scrub mitts can also be used to exfoliate the skin.

6. What are the harmful effects of exfoliating a little too much?

Exfoliating the skin more than once in a week can damage the protective barrier layer of the skin, making it sensitive and dry, and vulnerable to sun damage and infection. This leads to flaking, increased susceptibility to rashes and redness as well as premature aging in the form of fine lines, wrinkles and pigment spots. It can also lead to loss of suppleness, dull texture, itchiness and inflammatory acne.

7. What are the dos and don'ts of exfoliation?

The first thing to keep in mind is to exfoliate the skin gently. Always wet the skin first and then use the scrub or exfoliator. You should not scrub dry, flaky or irritated skin. It is best to stay away from scrubbing if you have any skin abrasions, infections, boils, pimples or pigmentation. Remember to moisturize your skin after exfoliating.

8. Why isn't an in-salon exfoliation always the best?

If a client has an existing viral infection such as molluscum contagiosum or humanpapilloma virus, both of which are contagious, it can be passed on to others visiting the salon. Folliculitis or hair follicle infection is another common problem when you exfoliate in salons. Moreover, if overdone, it can lead to pigmentation, rashes and sensitive skin.

9. Is lactic acid good for exfoliation? What is the percentage that can be used?

Lactic acid is an alpha hydroxy acid and is very mild. It is non-irritating and is derived from milk. You can use up to 10 per cent lactic acid very safely as a chemical exfoliant for sensitive skin or even dry skin.

10. Can I use a coffee scrub on my body if my skin is dry?

You can mix coffee powder with coconut or almond oil to scrub your body once a week. The almond oil or coconut oil will keep your skin hydrated while the coffee will help in gentle exfoliating. Make sure to apply a moisturizer on the body after you rinse the scrub off with water.

11. Can I exfoliate my underarms?

The underarm skin is very sensitive and exfoliating this area with a physical scrub is not advisable. Also, make sure that you do not use a high concentration of any acid because it may cause post-inflammatory hyperpigmentation or irritant contact dermatitis. You can use a polyhydroxy acid or a lactic acid serum to exfoliate the underarms.

12. I used 2 per cent salicylic acid for exfoliation, but it made my skin look duller and more tanned. What should I do?

You have probably over-exfoliated your skin. This deranges the barrier layer of the skin and rips the moisture away, making the skin look dry. Do not exfoliate anymore and avoid using soap-based body washes or shower gels. Instead, use a soap-free body wash and apply a moisturizer twice a day.

13. I am in my thirties and have sensitive skin. Is it okay to use AHA or BHA serum once in fifteen days?

It is better to avoid an AHA or a BHA serum since you have sensitive skin. You can use a polyhydroxy acid-based serum for mild chemical exfoliation.

14. What should be the sequence for cleansing, scrubbing, face mask and steam?

Doing all four of these together will be too much for the skin. You can steam your face, rinse with water and apply a face mask, or you can cleanse and apply a face mask, or you can scrub and apply a face mask. You should not steam and scrub your face at the same time because it will damage your skin, making it more dehydrated and sensitive.

15. Can I exfoliate my lips at home?

You can use yoghurt or malai, which is milk cream, mixed with a little sugar powder on the lips. Do not over-exfoliate the lips as the lip mucosa is unprotected and can be damaged easily, resulting in more cuts and chapped lips due to exfoliation.

16. What is a good scrub for combination skin?

You can use oatmeal mixed with honey and chickpea flour to gently exfoliate your face. Make sure not to over-exfoliate.

17. What strength of AHA and BHA can I use for chemical exfoliation at home?

Alpha hydroxy acids such as glycolic acid made of sugarcane extract, citric acid made of lemon extract and mandelic acid, which is from bitter almonds, are water-soluble, which means they cannot dissolve the oils in the skin. So, they are able to penetrate the stratum corneum, the dead skin layer, and exfoliate the dead skin. The concentrations that can be safely used at home should always be less than 10 per cent. Salicylic acid or beta hydroxy acid, which is a lipid-soluble acid, dissolves the oil or the sebum in the skin and helps unclog the pores. Again, the rule of thumb should be a concentration of less than 10 per cent if you are using it as a chemical exfoliant at home in the form of a serum or even a cream.

18. Is it okay to use a mixture of lemon, honey and coffee scrub on the face?

If you have sensitive, dry or combination skin, you have to be very careful with scrubs. You cannot use lemon as it can irritate the skin further and even cause burns. Honey can cause allergies and coffee won't really help the skin. Hence, it is better to avoid these ingredients individually or together if you have sensitive skin. If you have oily skin then you can use this combination once a week provided you are not using retinol, an alpha hydroxy acid, a beta hydroxy acid or an anti-acne cream that contains retinols or benzoyl peroxide.

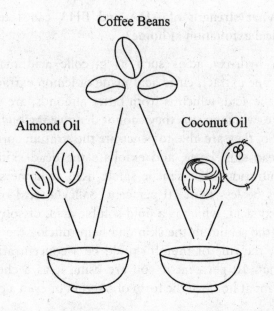

Coffee Beans

Almond Oil   Coconut Oil

19. Is 5 per cent glycolic acid safe to use during pregnancy?

Yes, glycolic acid is a sugarcane extract, and you can safely use up to 10 per cent of glycolic acid during pregnancy. Do not increase the concentration and make sure you do not apply it more than three times a week.

20. What is a good exfoliation method for hyperpigmentation?

When you have hyperpigmentation, it is better to avoid using mechanical scrubs, loofahs or pumice stones. This is because the friction will increase the chances of post-inflammatory hyperpigmentation, and it will also stimulate the pigment-forming cells to produce more melanin, thereby leading to an increase in pigmentation. You may use a chemical exfoliant such as an alpha hydroxy acid, for example glycolic acid, mandelic acid or lactic acid, twice or thrice a week. Make sure you always use a sunscreen from sunrise to sunset and also protect the skin from blue light which is emitted from cell phones, laptops and television screens.

21. Can we exfoliate with both a physical and chemical exfoliator at the same time?

While exfoliation is a good method to cleanse your skin, overdoing it can cause more damage than good. If you want to use a physical and chemical exfoliator, you must keep an interval of at least ten days between the two. If your skin feels irritated or becomes reddish you must stop exfoliation, give your skin some rest and then restart after three to four weeks with a very mild exfoliant such as a polyhydroxy acid or a lactic acid.

22. At what age should I start exfoliating my children's skin?

The skin has a normal twenty-eight-day cell cycle whereby the dead skin sheds on its own. Ideally exfoliation is not needed till this process slows down, which is usually when one is in their thirties. However, due to pollution, environmental impurities and unhealthy lifestyle the cell cycle may slow down, and a lot of dead skin may accumulate on the skin surface even in teenagers. So, exfoliate when their skin needs it.

RAPID FIRE

1. I play outdoors daily and sweat too much, should I be using a scrub to clean my face after my game?

You can just use a cleanser which removes all the dirt and sweat. Do not exfoliate daily.

2. Do I need to physically scrub my skin to cleanse it thoroughly?

Swap your fingertips for a physical scrub or loofah. They aren't really necessary.

3. Chemical exfoliants are all acids. What if they burn my skin?

Chemical exfoliants like AHAs and BHA available in the market are usually mild and don't cause harm if used judiciously.

4. I suffer from psoriasis. Should I exfoliate the flakes on my skin?

Absolutely not. Please do not use any physical or chemical exfoliant on your skin. You need to moisturize rather than exfoliate.

5. Can I use a mixture of crushed fruit to exfoliate my face?

It is best to avoid lest you want your skin to get irritated.

5

Moisturizers

'Moisturizer is to skin what water is to plants. Don't
neglect it.'

—Jaishree Sharad

The use of moisturizers to keep the skin soft and supple
dates back to 200 BC, when Cleopatra is said to have
used olive and palm oils on her skin to keep it youthful.
Australian aborigines used emu oil, made from a pad of
fat from the bird, to hydrate their skin. Galen, the Greek
physician, created the first cold cream: a mix of water,
olive oil, beeswax and floral oils in 150 AD. Petroleum
jelly was used for the first time in 1872 as a moisturizer
and ingredient in a lot of creams meant to hydrate the
skin. Indians have been using coconut oil and mustard oil
to massage the skin since decades as a customary skincare
ritual to keep the skin supple.

Moisturizing is an important part of a skincare routine and cannot be escaped. Let us understand why!

1. Why should I use a moisturizer?

The skin is the largest organ of the body. It shields the internal organs and protects the body from environmental toxins, pollution, microorganisms and harsh weather. However, the protective barrier layer of the skin can get compromised due to external aggressors such as pollution, ultraviolet rays, climate, stress, smoking or even products used on the skin. This can lead to dryness, eczema, allergies, acne, infections as well as early aging of skin. Thus, it is important to hydrate your skin internally by drinking water as well as externally by applying a moisturizer.

2. What are moisturizers?

Moisturizers are external agents that not only help increase the water content of the skin but also help

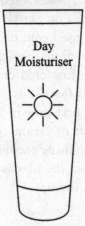

prevent water loss from the skin. These are available in cream, lotion and gel forms.

3. What are the types of moisturizers?

There are three types of moisturizers:

- Emollients, which spread all over the skin cells and moisturize the skin.
- Occlusives, which block the evaporation of water from the skin into the air.
- Humectants, which draw water from the deeper layers of the skin and from the environment and hydrate the skin by plumping the epidermis.

4. How do we choose the right moisturizer?

You can choose your moisturizer based on your skin type (dry, oily, combination or sensitive) and the climate. If you have oily skin, choose a water- or gel-based, non-comedogenic moisturizer. If you have dry skin, you need a cream-based moisturizer. If you have acne-prone skin, opt for a water-based moisturizer. If you have sensitive skin, you will need a moisturizer with minimal preservatives and no fragrance.

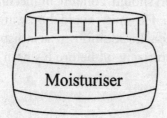

5. What are the benefits of moisturizers?

Moisturizers keep your skin hydrated. Well-hydrated skin looks healthy, soft, smooth, pliable and glowing. Moisturizing helps prevent dryness, itching and related diseases. Further, it helps reduce fine lines and the appearance of pores.

6. My grandfather has extremely dry skin and no moisturizer works for him. He scratches his skin all the time. You can literally write on his skin with your nails. Is there a solution to reduce this?

People above fifty years of age have much drier skin due to several changes in the skin. The upper epidermis becomes thin, the cell turnover reduces and the cell cycle slows down. The barrier layer of the skin is compromised as you age. As a result, there is more trans-epidermal water loss and the skin loses its ability to retain moisture. This is because the skin loses hyaluronic acid, which helps retain water in the skin. In females, the hormone oestrogen reduces, leading to skin dryness. As you age, the skin becomes more susceptible to environmental and climatic damage. Hence your grandfather and all those with mature and dry skin similar to his will need to apply a thick cream-based moisturizer at least three times a day. The moisturizer should contain humectants, occlusives and emollients. He must avoid hot water, scrubs and extreme climates. In addition to a moisturizer, he may also use a moisturizing oil before his bath and apply any oil once a day.

7. Can a moisturizer dry out skin?

Yes. Certain humectants such as lactic acid attract water and keep the skin hydrated. But in dry weather, they also tend to absorb water from the deeper layers of the skin, resulting in dryness. Hence one must use a moisturizer that contains both humectants and occlusives.

8. What should one avoid when choosing a moisturizer for the face?

If you want to buy a moisturizer without a dermatologist having prescribed one, it is better to avoid those with fragrance, synthetic dyes, astringents and alcohol because these ingredients are likely to cause allergic reactions.

9. When should I use a moisturizer?

Ideally, a moisturizer should be applied immediately after a bath when the skin is slightly moist. This helps lock in the moisture and retain it for a longer duration.

10. Does using a moisturizer regularly slow aging?

Yes, a moisturizer hydrates the skin and protects the barrier layer of the skin. This reduces inflammation, fights free radicals and helps slow down the process of aging. Besides, moisturizers with hyaluronic acid absorb and retain water, plumping the skin and making it look youthful.

11. I have oily skin; do I still need a moisturizer?

Even if you have oily skin, you need a moisturizer to keep your skin hydrated. Moisturizers add water to the skin

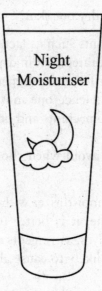

and help retain the water in the skin. Oily skin occurs due to excessive production of sebum by the oil glands. So, oily skin and hydrated skin are two different things. Opt for a water-based or a lightweight gel-based moisturizer. You may reduce the number of applications per day depending on your skin's requirement and the climate that you are in. Look for ingredients such as kaolin, dimethicone, hyaluronic acid and niacinamide which will moisturize your skin without clogging your pores or making the skin feel greasy.

12. Is Vaseline good for your face?

Vaseline contains petroleum jelly. It acts as an occlusive, which means it forms a barrier over the skin surface, prevents trans-epidermal water loss and maintains the moisture content of the skin. It may be a good option for people with more mature skin and those who have extremely dry skin. Those with oily or acne-prone skin should avoid petroleum jelly on the face as it can clog the pores, resulting in blackheads or whiteheads.

13. Can I use oils instead of moisturizing creams?

Oils are greasy. They lock the pores and sometimes even increase sebum production, resulting in acne, specially, if you have acne-prone skin. Hence use oils only if you have extremely dry skin. Those above the age of fifty who usually do not get acne can use oils on the face to moisturize their skin.

14. What is the most natural moisturizer?

Honey, aloe vera, olive oil, coconut oil, sunflower oil, shea butter and jojoba oil are all natural moisturizers. Oils are usually occlusives and should be used with caution if you have oily or acne-prone skin.

15. How can I hydrate my face?

Choose a good moisturizer as per your skin type and apply twice a day. During winter or if the skin feels very dry, you may apply a moisturizer more than twice. Avoid exfoliating your face frequently. Drink approximately 3 litres of water per day unless you have a medical condition where you are not supposed to drink too much water.

16. Should the day moisturizer be different from the night moisturizer?

If you have very dry skin, you may opt for the same moisturizer during the day and night. If you have normal, combination or oily skin, you can use a lightweight moisturizer in the morning and a thicker moisturizer that contains occlusives at bedtime.

17. How do you rehydrate aging skin?

Regular use of moisturizer helps keep the skin hydrated but with increasing age the skin becomes thin, and its moisture-retaining capacity decreases. So, repeated application is needed. Hyaluronic acid injections known as skin boosters help improve skin quality and reduce dryness.

18. Can a face moisturizer be used for the body and vice versa?

Face moisturizers are usually lighter than body moisturizers. Besides, the skin type of the face and body are not always the same. So, a face moisturizer may not work for the body and vice versa.

19. Should I keep changing my moisturizer?

Yes, you may need to change your moisturizer depending on your skin type, climate, the temperatures you are exposed to during the day, your existing skin condition, the products you use on a daily basis, right from cleansers to medicated creams, the medicines you take and your hormones.

20. Can I use the same moisturizer in summer and winter?

The moisture content of one's skin varies as per the weather and climatic conditions. In winter the skin becomes dry, hence you need to apply a heavy moisturizer with an occlusive and emulsifying effect. In summer, as sweating increases trans-epidermal water loss, you need water- or gel-based moisturizers instead of oily moisturizers or those with a humectant and occlusive effect. Similarly, if you travel to places where the temperature is low and it is cold, you will need a heavier moisturizer than in a place that is hot or humid.

21. Can I use moisturizers with SPF or do I have to use both products separately?

If you are indoors all day long you may use a moisturizer with SPF but if you have to step outdoors, you will need a moisturizer and a sunscreen in addition to it. A moisturizer with SPF is never enough when you are outdoors.

22. Can I skip a moisturizer and just use a serum?

Serums are concentrated forms of solutions with active ingredients. They may not possess the emollient effect of a moisturizer. Hence you should not skip using a moisturizer. You should apply the serum and then apply a moisturizer over it.

23. I develop acne with moisturizers. But my face gets dry at times. What should I do?

You need to apply a moisturizer that is non-comedogenic, non-greasy and water- or gel-based. Ceramide-based moisturizers are best for acne-prone skin as they help reduce inflammation and protect the skin from further damage.

24. Do oral moisturizers work?

Oral moisturizers contain ceramosides, a patented complex of plant ceramides. They are said to increase ceramide content in the skin when taken orally. Ceramosides are said to have anti-inflammatory, antioxidant, collagen-boosting and hydrating properties. However, adequate research is lacking.

25. Why is my moisturizer not working?

You could be using the wrong moisturizer or the wrong combination of skincare products with your moisturizer. Using the same moisturizer in all seasons and using a fragrance-based moisture could be other reasons why it is not working for you. Also, make sure that you are not rubbing your moisturizer vigorously into the skin.

26. I have extremely dry skin. What ingredients should I look for in my moisturizer?

You should use a combination of humectants, occlusives and emollients. Humectants such as hyaluronic acid, sorbitol, proteins, panthenol, urea, glycerine and propylene glycol help attract water to your skin. Occlusives such as petrolatum, lanolin, silicon, beeswax, vegetable oil (for example, coconut oil, castor oil, olive oil, grape seed oil and soybean oil) and mineral oil help lock in moisture. Emollients such as cholesterol, fatty acids, ceramides, fatty alcohol and squalene hydrate the skin.

27. What are ceramides?

Ceramides comprise 30 to 40 per cent of the lipids in the stratum corneum, that is, the uppermost layers of our skin. Ceramides offer many benefits for the skin. They can improve the health of the skin cells, help create a barrier to prevent moisture from leaving the skin, prevent dryness and irritation by locking moisture into the skin, protect the skin from environmental damage, protect the skin from allergy and infection-causing germs like bacteria and fungi, and promote anti-aging by keeping the skin moist and supple.

28. Does everybody need moisturizers with ceramides?

No. Ceramides are necessary for those with compromised barrier function of the skin. So, people with extremely dry skin or conditions such as atopic dermatitis, psoriasis, acne or ichthyosis require ceramides in their moisturizer in order to rebuild the protective barrier layer in the skin.

29. How do we know if ceramides are present in our moisturizer?

There are twelve types of ceramides, named ceramide 1 to 12. They are usually listed on the labels of skincare products as: Ceramide 1, also called ceramide EOS; Ceramide 2, also called ceramide NS or NG; Ceramide 3, also called ceramide NP; Ceramide 6-II, also called ceramide AP; Ceramide 9, also called ceramide EOP; phytosphingosine; and sphingosine.

RAPID FIRE

1. Can we apply sunscreen after applying moisturizer?

Most certainly. A sunscreen should always be applied over a moisturizer during the day.

2. Is a moisturizer with SPF enough on the beach?

Not at all. Always use a separate moisturizer and sunscreen with SPF 50 and PA 4+ when you are on the beach.

3. Should one not apply a moisturizer in summer?

You should moisturize 365 days a year.

4. Is moisturizer mandatory for oily, acne-prone skin?

Yes, acne-prone skin needs ceramides as moisturizing ingredients in the skin.

5. Can we use aloe vera gel we get at the chemist as a moisturizer?

Only if you have very oily skin and your skin in not sensitive.

6. I use a water-based moisturizer for extremely dry acne-prone skin, but my skin still feels dry.

Use a moisturizer with ceramides in it.

7. Should one moisturize after washing hands?

Always.

8. How many times a day should I apply moisturizer on my face?

Minimum once and as often as your skin feels dry.

9. How can I remove dryness from my face?

Use a gentle, soap-free cleanser. Apply a thick moisturizer with emollient and occlusive properties. Drink plenty of water.

10. Can all of us at home use the same body lotion?

Only if all of you have the same skin type.

6

Sunscreens

'We all need that one best friend who stands by us in good times and bad. A sunscreen is that best friend for your skin.'

—Jaishree Sharad

A sunscreen is an essential skincare product which should be used 365 days of the year.

4000 BC: Egyptians were the first civilization to use the extracts of rice bran, jasmine and lupine to block the tanning effect of the sun where rice absorbs UV light, jasmine repairs DNA and lupine lightens the skin

In 600 BC, athletes used olive oil and fine sand to protect their skin from the sun's drying rays. Later, olive oil was confirmed to have an SPF rating of 8.

Sunscreen Recommendations (quoted from J. Tsai, and A.L. Chien, A.L. Photoprotection for Skin of Color. *American Journal of Clinical Dermatology* 23, 195–205 (2022). https://doi.org/10.1007/s40257-021-00670-z

Pushpanjan or zinc oxide which is now used in all physical sunscreens was discovered in the *Charaka Samhita,* an ancient Indian medical literature in 500 BC.

The first chemical sunscreen was formulated in 1891 by a German scientist Friedrich Hammer by using acidified quinine sulphate in lotion and ointment which reduced the UVB-induced sunburn effect.

Current sunscreen recommendations as quoted from the *American Journal of Clinical Dermatology* are to apply a broad-spectrum sunscreen of about 2 mg/cm^2 with SPF 30 or higher. Make sure to apply it fifteen minutes before sun exposure and then reapply every two hours. Tinted sunscreens and sunscreens based on non-micronized inorganic filters are preferred for protection against both UV radiation and visible light, and sunscreens with nano-sized inorganic filters or organic filters are suitable options if transparent formulations are desired, but they protect against UV radiation and not visible light. Along with this, wear a hat, sunglasses and sun-protective clothing (e.g., long-sleeved shirt, pants) with a UPF of 30 or higher and seek shade and avoid sun exposure during peak daylight hours, that is, 10 a.m. to 4 p.m.

1. What exactly are sunrays made up of?

Solar radiation comprises ultraviolet (UV) rays, visible light and infrared rays. UV rays that reach the earth's surface comprise UVA (320–400 nm wavelength) and UVB (290–320 nm wavelength) rays. Visible rays are at about 400–800 nm wavelength, infrared rays are anything above 800 nm wavelength. Wavelengths of less than 320 nm are absorbed by the upper layer of the skin, namely, the stratum corneum and epidermis.

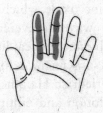

The amount of sunscreen you can apply to your face

Wavelengths greater than 320 nm enter the deeper part of the skin, the dermis. All rays cause the breakdown of cell membranes, lipids, structural proteins and DNA of the skin. UVA and UVB rays can cause rashes, allergies like polymorphous light eruptions and hyperpigmentation. UVA rays penetrate the deeper layers of the skin (dermis) and can cause age spots or liver spots, premature aging of skin, wrinkles, fine lines, enlarged pores, solar elastosis, uneven skin tone and tanning. UVA rays are known to generate reactive oxygen species and alter the DNA and connective tissue. This leads to immunosuppression as well. UVB rays, on the other hand, penetrate the upper layers of the skin (epidermis) and can cause sunburn and actinic keratoses (dry rough patch of skin which may turn cancerous). Prolonged exposure to UVB rays can also result in skin cancer. Infrared rays and visible light can also penetrate the deeper layers of the skin and cause effects similar to those caused by UVA rays.

2. Is sunscreen essential and why?

Yes, sunscreen is essential. It protects you from the harmful effects of UVA and UVB rays, visible light and blue light. The ozone layer in the atmosphere is depleting, and the body needs protection from all the harmful rays.

3. Who needs to wear sunscreen?

Anyone above the age of six months irrespective of gender, race or age needs to apply a sunscreen every single day.

4. What are SPF and PA?

SPF or sun protection factor is defined as the ratio of the time of UV exposure necessary to produce minimally detectable erythema in sunscreen-protected skin to that time for unprotected skin. The SPF value denotes how many more times the skin is protected against ultraviolet rays after using sunscreen. For example, if unprotected skin's minimal erythema dose is ten minutes, when a sunscreen with SPF 30 is applied, the skin will be protected for 300 minutes. PA value is the protection from UVA rays. PA+ means low protection, PA++ is moderate, PA+++ is high and PA++++ is very high UVA protection.

5. Isn't SPF 100 better than SPF 30 or SPF 50?

A sunscreen with SPF 15 blocks 93 per cent of UVB radiation, SPF 30 blocks 97 per cent, SPF 50 blocks 98 per cent and SPF 100 blocks 99 per cent of UVB rays from reaching your skin. So, there isn't a significant difference between SPF 30 and SPF 100. It is best to apply SPF 50 when one is outdoors or on the beach or in the mountains or snow.

S. Levy Sunscreens. In S. Wolverton, editor. *Comprehensive Dermatologic Drug Therapy*. 3rd ed. Philadelphia: Saunders, 2012, p. 551–61. Back to cited text no. 8

6. How do we select a sunscreen?

Your sunscreen will depend on your skin type (dry, oily, acne-prone or sensitive); the number of hours you spend outdoors in the sun; your skin condition such as hyperpigmentation, rosacea, acne, sun, allergies, etc.; and the climate that you are exposed to. Always opt for a broad-spectrum sunscreen that protects the skin from both UVA and UVB rays. These days sunscreens also contain iron oxide, botanicals and antioxidants, which protect the skin from infrared rays, visible light and blue light as well. If you have oily or acne-prone skin, you will need a water-based, gel-based or matte sunscreen that will not make the skin greasy. A non-comedogenic sunscreen will not clog your pores and will not increase blackheads and whiteheads. If you have dry skin, you can use a cream-based sunscreen preferably with moisturizing ingredients such as hyaluronic acid, ceramides or dimethicone to keep your skin hydrated. If you have sensitive skin, opt for a mineral sunscreen. If you have sun allergies or hyperpigmentation or you are going to spend longer hours in the sun, you need a sunscreen with an SPF of at least 50 and PA++++. Use a sunscreen that is fragrance-free in order to avoid sun-induced allergies and hyperpigmentation. And always look for the date of manufacture and date of expiry of the sunscreen.

7. Is applying sunscreen enough to protect the skin from UV rays?

In addition to applying sunscreen, one should also wear clothing that covers the arms and legs, wide-brimmed hats and UV-protective sunglasses when exposed to direct sunlight. An umbrella is also a good option. UV-protective clothing is excellent for those prone to skin cancer. Avoid stepping outdoors between 10 a.m. and 4 p.m., when sunrays are the strongest. You can also take supplements of vitamin C, superoxide dismutase or polypodium leucotomos, which act as oral sunscreens, protecting the skin from the harmful effects of UV rays by fighting the free radicals which develop in the skin upon sun exposure (they don't replace a topical sunscreen, though).

8. What is the correct method of using sunscreen?

The current US Food and Drug Administration standard recommends 2 mg/cm² of skin surface. For the face and neck, apply ½ teaspoon (3 ml) of sunscreen. Apply ½ teaspoon (3 ml) of sunscreen on each arm. Apply 1 teaspoon (6 ml) of sunscreen on each leg, and 1 teaspoon on both feet. Apply 1 teaspoon of sunscreen on the chest and 2 teaspoons on the entire back. Remember to apply sunscreen on the back of your neck, ears and hairline.

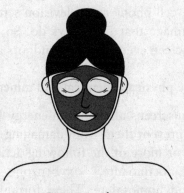

Sunscreen face

The other simple rule is the two-finger rule. This means that two strips of sunscreen should be squeezed from the base to the tip of the middle and index fingers and applied to the entire face.

9. Should one apply sunscreen on cloudy days?

Seventy-five to 80 per cent of UVA rays penetrate clouds easily and can even reach below the water's surface. Hence it is important to apply sunscreen even on cloudy days and even when you are in the pool or seawater.

10. Can I skip the sunscreen in my skincare routine since I do not step out of my house at all during the day?

Seventy-five per cent of UVA rays penetrate glass. So, glass windows at home or in your office or the glass windows of your car cannot shield you from UVA rays, visible light and infrared rays. Besides, there may be times when you step out on to your balcony or go to your terrace or just sip coffee by the window, thus exposing your skin to these rays. Not only that, the blue light from your laptop, cell phone and television screens can cause the same damage that UVA rays do. So, it is better to apply a sunscreen even if you are indoors all the time.

11. What are physical, chemical and mineral sunscreens?

Chemical sunscreens absorb high-energy UV rays like a sponge and prevent them from damaging the skin. They contain one or more of the following active ingredients: octocrylene, octinoxate, oxybenzone, avobenzone, octisalate and homosalate. These formulations do not leave a white residue on the skin and are easier to rub into the skin.

Physical sunscreens work like a shield, sitting on the surface of the skin and deflecting the sun's rays. They contain the active ingredients zinc oxide and/or titanium dioxide. However, they may leave a white residue on the skin.

Newer formulations with micronized particles are better, and do not leave an opaque cast. They are also known as mineral sunscreens and are safe options for children, pregnant women and people with sensitive skin.

Broad-spectrum sunscreens protect the skin from UVA and UVB rays. They may contain both physical and chemical sunscreen ingredients in them. Ingredients such as Mexoryl, ecamsule, tinosorb M, etc. are broad-spectrum. Some sunscreens contain antioxidants such as vitamin C, vitamin E, silymarin and green tea polyphenols for added protection against UVA and UVB rays and for protection against visible and blue light.

Tinted sunscreens are best for those with exposure to harsh camera lights or blue light from laptop screens. The tint is achieved by incorporating a blend of iron oxides and pigmentary titanium dioxide. Iron oxide is known to protect the skin from blue light. Those suffering from hyperpigmentation such as melasma or blue light induced dermatoses should use tinted sunscreens.

12. Is sunscreen advisable while playing as sweat rubs off the sunscreen?

Yes, it is important to use sunscreen especially when you are out in the sun, whether you are playing a game or watching one, in order to prevent hyperpigmentation. You must have seen cricketers wear a white paste on their face while playing. That is a physical sunblock. Sweat-resistant sunscreen, which is supposed to protect you for up to forty to eighty minutes of continuous heavy perspiration, is a good option too. You can even apply two fingers of a waterproof physical sunblock and layer it with talc for added protection. Some of the sunblock may get rubbed off with sweat. But it is better than no sun protection at all. If you can reapply, nothing better.

13. Should one apply sunscreen when swimming?

A combination of chlorine and sunlight can be detrimental to the skin. It is extremely important to apply a sunscreen if you are swimming in broad daylight in an outdoor pool. Opt for a water-resistant or waterproof sunscreen and apply it fifteen minutes before you step into the pool because it takes approximately fifteen minutes for the sunscreen to get absorbed into the skin. A water-resistant sunscreen protects the skin for up to forty minutes in the water.

14. Doesn't sunscreen prevent the synthesis of vitamin D in the body?

The American Academy of Dermatology says that the amount of vitamin D a person receives from the sun is inconsistent and excessive sun exposure in order to obtain vitamin D increases the risk of skin cancer. It is better to obtain vitamin D from foods naturally rich in

---

American Academy of Dermatology Association, 'Sunscreen FAQ', https://www.aad.org/media/stats-sunscreen

vitamin D, foods and beverages fortified with vitamin D, and/or vitamin D supplements.

15. Do I need to apply a sunscreen if my screen time is more?

Almost 50 per cent of the sunlight spectrum consists of light that is visible to the naked eye, called visible light. It has a wavelength ranging from 400 nm to 760 nm. The wavelength between 400 nm to 500 nm is known as blue light or high-energy visible light. This blue light can also be emitted by your television, computer, laptop and mobile phone screens. Blue light can increase the amount of DNA damage and cell and tissue death, leading to early signs of aging such as fine lines, wrinkles and sagging as well as hyperpigmentation.

So yes, you do need to apply a sunscreen even if you remain indoors 24x7. Iron oxide, vitamin C, botanicals, antioxidants, etc. protect us from blue light. Look for these ingredients in your sunscreen or opt for tinted sunscreens. Tinted sunscreens contain varied amounts of iron oxide and pigmentary titanium dioxide, which protect us from blue light.

16. Are there any side effects of sunscreen?

Sunscreen ingredients such as PABA, aminobenzoic acid and oxybenzone as well as fragrance can cause contact dermatitis or photosensitivity reactions. These ingredients should be avoided to prevent side effects such as redness, itching of the skin and stinging of the eyes. You can opt instead for mineral sunscreens. Serious allergic reactions are rare; however, if you notice any side effects, check with your dermatologist.

17. Do sunscreens cause cancer?

Sunscreens protect us from developing skin cancer as they protect us from the harmful effects of UVB rays. Benzene, which is supposed to be cancer-causing, was found as a contaminant in certain sunscreens and is not a sunscreen ingredient per se. Sunscreens containing benzene as a contaminant have been withdrawn from the market. According to the American Academy of Dermatology, in 2019, the US Food and Drug Administration announced that it would re-evaluate the safety of every ingredient used in chemical sunscreens to determine whether their absorption into the bloodstream had any effects on a person's health. (Just because an ingredient is absorbed into the bloodstream does not mean that it is harmful or unsafe.) The Food and Drug Administration continues to advise consumers to use sunscreen to protect themselves from the sun's dangerous UV rays.

18. Does a sunscreen mixed with a moisturizer lower the protective factor?

A sunscreen mixed with moisturizer may not have the efficacy that a sunscreen alone can have. Also, you should use at least half a teaspoon of the product on the entire face with reapplication every two hours. Using a sunscreen mixed with moisturizer can therefore be inconvenient and make your face greasy. Hence it is better to use a sunscreen separately.

19. Should I wash my face every time I reapply sunscreen?

Ideally, it is better to wash your face every time you want to reapply sunscreen, but it may not be practical.

Instead, you can spray some thermal water mist on your face, dab your skin with a tissue and then reapply the sunscreen.

20. My dermatologist advised me not to use sunscreen often as it can lead to acne. Is that true?

If your sunscreen is cream-based and contains a lot of comedogenic ingredients, it can lead to acne. However, there are many sunscreens that are non-comedogenic and can be used even if you have acne-prone skin.

21. I work the night shift. Should I apply sunscreen on my face while working on my laptop?

Blue light from the laptop screen can harm the skin as much as UVA. Use a blue light filter on your laptop or apply a physical sunscreen that contains zinc oxide and titanium dioxide along with antioxidants such as vitamins C and E, and plant extracts (phenolic, carotenoids and flavonoid compounds), which will protect you from blue light. Iron oxide is a great ingredient to look out for in your sunscreen for that added protection from blue light and infrared rays. Most tinted sunscreens would contain iron oxide.

22. What kind of sunscreen should one use for dry skin?

Opt for a sunscreen that has additional moisturizing ingredients such as ceramides, hyaluronic acid, vitamin E, etc. as these will keep the skin moisturized.

23. I have oily, acne-prone skin and sunscreen makes my skin oilier. What should I do ?

You need to opt for sunscreens that are matte or gel- or water-based. Matte sunscreens absorb oil and prevent the skin from looking oily. Gel- or water-based sunscreens are lightweight and non-greasy, and their formulations are suitable for oily or acne-prone skin. They do not leave a white cast on the skin surface.

24. At what age should a child start applying sunscreen?

A sunscreen can be applied on a child over six months old. Sunscreens for children usually do not contain chemical ingredients. Fragrance-free, paraben-free, mineral formulations with UVA and UVB blocking ingredients such as zinc oxide and titanium dioxide are safe for kids. Look for labels that say paediatric, safe for children or kids' sunscreen.

25. How many times a day should I apply sunscreen?

The effect of the best of sunscreens wears off in two to three hours. Hence one must reapply a sunscreen every two to three hours when outdoors, however high the SPF or the PA may be and however expensive or reputed the sunscreen may be.

26. What is the difference between a cream or lotion and spray sunscreen?

Sunscreens come in various formulations. A cream is easy to apply on smaller areas while lotions, having higher spreadability, can be applied on larger areas. Stick sunscreens are also popular when you are travelling or when you are outdoors and need to reapply the sunscreen. Sprays are most convenient when you need to reapply the sunscreen on larger surface areas. However, you will have to spray a lot more sunscreen than a cream or lotion as it is difficult to measure quantity when you are using a spray. Also, sprays result in uneven spreading of sunscreen agents.

27. My skin tans quickly even after applying a sunscreen. What should I do?

First of all, you need to choose a broad-spectrum sunscreen with an SPF of at least 30 and PA+++. Do not forget to use a two-finger quantity on the entire face. Reapply the sunscreen every two hours when you're outdoors. Wear UV-protective dark glasses, clothing that covers your arms and legs, and a wide-brimmed hat or a scarf in addition to the sunscreen. Sunscreens may not protect you from visible light and blue light if they do not contain blue light and visible light protecting ingredients. Take supplements of vitamins C and E as well as antioxidants to protect you further from the sun's rays.

28. My skin turns darker when I apply a sunscreen. Should I avoid using one?

If your sunscreen contains photosensitizing ingredients such as certain fragrances like bergamot oil, lemon oil, geraniol, and hydroxycitronellal, musk, etc., or sometimes a high concentration of a chemical ingredient such as oxybenzone, it may cause further darkening of skin upon sun exposure. Certain salts of vitamin C such as L ascorbic acid that are easily oxidized on sun exposure should also be avoided in your sunscreen. Hence opt for sunscreens that are fragrance-free and do not contain oxidizing or photosensitizing agents.

29. Why does one need to apply sunscreen every day?

A sunscreen protects you from UVA and UVB rays, visible light, infrared rays as well as blue light, which not only comes from the sun but also from your laptop, cell phone and television screens. These rays can cause hyperpigmentation, early signs of aging and even allergies. Thus you should use sunscreen every day whether indoors or outdoors, whether it's sunny or cloudy, whether you're in the hills or at the beach.

30. Do I need a sunscreen when it's snowing and temperatures are very low?

Snow can reflect almost 90 per cent of UV radiation. This means that you can be exposed to almost a double dose of UV directly from the sun and bouncing off snow-covered surfaces. Thus it is mandatory to use a sunscreen with SPF 50 and PA+++ even when it's snowing, and to make sure to reapply it every two to three hours.

31. I'm visiting a hill station for my holidays and it will be really cold. Should I still be wearing a sunscreen?

The atmosphere is thinner and there is less pollution to filter out UV rays at higher altitudes such as the mountains. UV radiation intensity increases by about 10 to 12 per cent for every 1000-metre increase in altitude. Thus you need a sunscreen when you're in the mountains too even though it may be pleasant and cool. To add to this, if there is snow you need added UV protection, as snow reflects UV rays.

32. What kind of clothes should one wear to protect the skin from UV rays ?

Bright or dark colours absorb UV rays and prevent them from reaching the skin. Hence they give you better protection than light shades even when your skin is entirely covered. Satins, silks and shiny polyesters reflect rays and protect the skin. Some special fabrics even have ultraviolet protection factor (UPF) and are best suited for outdoor activities, especially for those with fairer skin or if you are engaging in outdoor activities for several hours and the risk of skin cancer is high. Loose-fitting clothes are better than tight-fitted clothes when it comes to UV protection. The fibres of tight-fitting clothes get stretched, allowing more UV rays to pass through. Wet clothes also offer less UV protection. Last but not the least, the more skin your clothes cover the better the protection.

33. What is UPF?

Ultraviolet protection factor (UPF) indicates how much UV radiation (both UVA and UVB) a fabric allows to reach your skin. A UPF 50 fabric blocks 98 per cent of the sun's rays and allows 2 per cent to penetrate the skin. A UPF of 30 to 49 offers very good sun protection while UPF 50+ gives excellent UV protection.

34. I have a sunburn on my forehead and whenever I go outside, I put a sunscreen with an SPF value of 50, but the area is very itchy and I now have a dry patch there.

I have tried applying neem leaves and aloe vera. Nothing works. What should I do?

You seem to be suffering from a sun allergy or some form of contact dermatitis. You will need to apply a medicated cream on the itchy patch at bedtime. During the day, you must apply a moisturizer followed by a sunscreen. Do consult a dermatologist instead of trying home remedies.

35. I am going on a beach holiday. My skin is very sensitive and tans easily. I want to prevent tanning and breakouts. What regime should I follow?

Water, sand and snow reflect UV rays, thereby causing more harm to the skin. Exposure to the sun while on the beach can cause severe tanning, sunburn and allergic reactions, while delayed effects can include pigmentation, sunspots, fine lines and wrinkles. The skin is more prone to sunburn in the midday sun. So, plan to go to the beach before 10 a.m. or after 4 p.m., as the sun's rays are less intense during this period. Water-resistant sunscreens protect the skin for forty minutes of water exposure. Some water-resistant sunscreens protect for up to eighty minutes. Apply a water-resistant sunscreen lotion with SPF 50 about fifteen minutes before getting into seawater. After a swim or plunge in the sea, make sure to moisturize your skin as well as lips to prevent peeling and drying of the skin. Cocoa or shea butter is the best bet. Wear sunglasses that protect against UVA and UVB rays. Wear a hat with a wide brim as it provides additional sun protection for your face and hair. You can also use an umbrella and scarf.

Keep yourself hydrated by drinking plenty of water, coconut water or other fruit juices. Have a great holiday!

36. I am in my twenties and my job involves a lot of travelling. The summer is worrying me as my skin becomes splotchy and uneven due to overexposure to the sun. How can I deal with this?

Carry a sunscreen with you at all times. Apply a sunscreen with SPF 30 and PA++++ at least 15 minutes before you step outdoors in order to allow the sunscreen to get absorbed into the skin completely. Your sunscreen should be both UVA and UVB protective. If you are out in the sun for more than three hours, you must reapply the sunscreen as it will photodegrade or get rubbed off in three hours no matter how expensive or good it may be. Try to carry an umbrella or wear a wide-brimmed hat or at least tie a scarf to protect your face. Oral sunscreens, vitamin C and antioxidant supplements also help.

37. Whenever I use a sunscreen, my face becomes greasy, and I start perspiring. When I am forced to wipe my face, the sunscreen comes off too. Since I have a field job, please guide me on how to prevent a suntan.

Use a sunscreen that contains zinc oxide or titanium dioxide. These are physical sunblocks and they stay on in spite of sweating. Dust a little loose powder on the sunscreen. However, if you wipe your face, you need to reapply the sunscreen. Wear wide-rimmed dark glasses and carry an umbrella too. Drink plenty of water to keep yourself well hydrated. Avoid the sun between 10 a.m. and 4 p.m.

38. My eyes sting every time I apply sunscreen under the eyes. Should I avoid sunscreen in this area? I have hyperpigmentation under my eyes.

Some sunscreens may sting if applied very close to the eyes. This is due to fragrance, or certain preservatives or chemical filters in the sunscreen. Opt for fragrance-free, physical or mineral sunscreens in such situations.

39. What are oral sunscreens?

Vitamins A, C and E, lycopene, green tea polyphenols and selenium are potent antioxidants that protect the skin from free radical damage than can occur with UVA, infrared and visible light.

Another popular oral sunscreen is polypodium leucotomos (PL), a fern that is native to South America. It contains a natural mixture of phytochemicals with powerful antioxidant and photoprotective properties. One capsule is recommended thirty minutes before stepping out in the sun

RAPID FIRE

1. Is it necessary to reapply sunscreen after having applied it once in the morning?

Sunscreens should be reapplied approximately every two hours when outdoors, even on cloudy days, and after sweating or swimming. The most efficacious sunscreens

S. Tahiliani and M. Shirolikar Viva Voce on Sunscreens. *Indian Journal of Drugs Dermatology* [serial online] 2018 [cited 2022 July 31], 4:92–96.

will also become photodegraded or rubbed off after two to three hours.

2. Do I have to apply sunscreen on skin covered by clothing, such as on the thighs?

If your clothing covers your arms and legs and is made of fabric that shields you from UVA and UVB rays, then you need not apply a sunscreen to those areas.

3. I am allergic to fragrance and have sensitive skin. Can you suggest a suitable sunscreen?

You need to opt for a fragrance-free, hypoallergenic, paraben-free, chemical-free sunscreen. Mineral sunscreens that contain ingredients such as zinc oxide and titanium dioxide are safe options.

4. Should I apply sunscreen or regular cream first on my face?

Always use a sunscreen over your day cream or moisturizer, right before you apply make-up. For more, refer to the chapter on layering of skincare products.

5. Is the SPF in compact powder or spray form equally effective as that of a normal sunscreen?

Compact powder may not be as effective as a cream- or gel-based sunscreen, but it can certainly be used for touch-up over make-up when one is outdoors.

6. Can one use sunscreen during pregnancy ?

Indeed, opt for a fragrance-free, mineral sunscreen.

7. I work in a closed office which has glass walls and travel by car to my office. Do I still need a sunscreen ?

Yes, 70 per cent of UVA penetrates glass, whether they are walls or car windows.

8. Should I apply sunscreen to my two-year-old?

Yes, apply a a pediatric sunscreen to the exposed parts of the body fifteen minutes before you take him outdoors.

9. I trek in dense forests where there is no direct sunlight. I walk in the shade. Do I still need a sunscreen ?

Whenever there is daylight, irrespective of direct or indirect sun exposure, you need a sunscreen.

10. I hate applying creams on my skin. Can I skip the sunscreen and take some oral supplements instead?

There is no substitute for a topical sunscreen. Although there are some oral sunscreens available, their efficacy hasn't been proven. Besides, oral sunscreens do not provide full protection from UVA and UVB rays.

7

Active Ingredients

'Be selective about your life goals, your friends and your skincare.'

—Jaishree Sharad

The history of active ingredients such as alpha hydroxy acids dates back 3000 years when Cleopatra, the ancient Egyptian queen, supposedly bathed in sour milk every day to improve the colour and texture of her skin. Sour milk contains lactic acid, an alpha hydroxy acid. The ancient Egyptians also used animal oils, salt and alabaster to improve the skin. Poultices containing mustard, sulfur, corrosive sublimate of limestone, fermented grape juice, soured milk, wine and lemon extract were used later by the Greeks and the Romans to lighten and brighten their skin. Grape juice and wine contain tartaric acid and lemon extract contains citric acid, both of which are alpha hydroxy acids. Retinol was used to treat conditions like xerosis and follicular hyperkeratosis (dry skin and thickening of skin around hair follicles respectively) during World War I. Active ingredients have been a part of the dermatologists arsenal since years.

It is important to choose the right ingredient and the right skincare product which will target your skin concern without giving you side effects. Here, I have all your queries on active ingredients answered in order to help you choose your product wisely.

ALPHA HYDROXY ACIDS

1. What are alpha hydroxy acids?

Alpha hydroxy acids (AHAs) are a group of natural acids derived from foods. They include citric acid (found in citrus fruits), glycolic acid (found in sugarcane), lactic acid (found in sour milk and tomato juice), malic acid (found in apples), tartaric acid (found in grapes) and mandelic acid (found in bitter almonds).

2. What do AHAs do?

Alpha hydroxy acids help in chemo exfoliation. They cause exfoliation of the superficial dead cell layers of the skin, leaving the skin texture smooth and helping in the reduction of superficial pigmentation. They are also known to boost collagen, firm the skin as well as improve fine lines and dilated pores. They may result in dryness in higher concentration, thereby neutralizing oil secretion, and can be used to reduce acne and post-acne blemishes.

Lactic acid, which is obtained from milk, also has moisturizing properties.

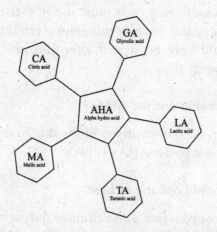

3. What concentration of AHA should be used?

The US Food and Drug Administration (FDA)-recommended concentration of AHAs in skincare products is less than 10 per cent.

4. Who can use AHAs?

AHAs are available in the form of serums, creams and lotions, and in higher concentrations, they are available as chemical peels, but these should only be administered in clinics. AHA serums can be used by those who want an even skin tone, improvement in acne spots, reduction in post-inflammatory hyperpigmentation, smooth skin texture, radiant skin, reduced pore size and improvement in fine lines.

5. Are AHAs suitable for all skin types?

No, AHAs are not suitable for all skin types. Those with normal, oily or combination skin can use AHAs regularly.

If you have dry skin, you must use it sparingly. If you have very dry and sensitive skin, please refrain from using it. It should only be started after guidance from your dermatologist.

6. When should one use AHAs?

AHAs increase the sensitivity of the skin to the sun hence it's important to use AHAs at night.

7. How should one use AHAs?

First, cleanse your face with a cleanser and pat it completely dry. Then apply three to five drops of the AHA serum on your face. Apply it at night so your skin doesn't become photosensitive. Initially, use an AHA twice a week and eventually, when your skin starts adapting well to the AHA, you can increase the frequency to thrice a week or even daily.

8. At what age can one use AHAs?

Whenever one sees signs of sun-induced pigmentation, textural changes in the skin, uneven skin tone or post-acne blemishes, usually after the age of sixteen, one can start using AHAs under the guidance of a dermatologist. We usually recommend AHAs for anti-aging at the age of twenty-five and above as part of the skincare routine.

9. Who should not use AHAs?

Those who have had an allergic reaction to any of the AHAs should refrain from using them. Avoid using AHAs immediately after bleaching your face, a chemical peel or Laser procedure. Do not use an AHA if the skin is extremely sensitive, peeling, or flaky and dry.

10. What are the side effects of AHAs?

Some people can develop redness, burning and irritation after using products containing AHAs. Opt for lactic acid serum, which is milder, if your skin is unable to tolerate glycolic acid, which is among the stronger AHAs.

11. What should you not combine an AHA with?

Avoid layering AHAs with retinol, vitamin C or beta hydroxy acid (BHA) at the same time as they may cause extreme exfoliation and rashes. You may apply an AHA on one night and a retinol the other night or a BHA on one night and a retinol on the other night while you can use vitamin C in the day.

12. How does one choose which AHA to use?

If you have dry skin or are undergoing an acne treatment that causes exfoliation, opt for lactic acid, which has skin-lightening as well as hydrating properties. Mandelic acid is a good option if you have acne and post-acne blemishes. For mature skin above the age of thirty, when the skin type is normal or oily, one can use glycolic acid.

13. What are beta hydroxy acids?

Beta hydroxy acids (BHAs) are most commonly available as salicylic acid. Salicylic acid is obtained from wintergreen leaves, willow bark or sweet birch.

14. Who should use salicylic acid?

Those with normal, oily, combination or acne-prone skin can use salicylic acid-based face washes or up to 10 per cent salicylic acid-based serums. Those with dry or sensitive skin should not use a BHA serum.

Salicylic acid is lipophilic, which means it is lipid-soluble. It penetrates deeper into the skin, dissolves sebum and unclogs pores. BHAs help reduce acne, blackheads, whiteheads, clogged pores and seborrhoea. They are chemo exfoliants hence also help reduce post-acne blemishes and hyperpigmentation.

15. Who should not be using BHAs?

If you are pregnant or planning pregnancy, you should avoid using BHAs. Also, those who have had allergies to any BHAs should refrain from using salicylic acid. If your skin is excessively dry and flaky, or if you are undergoing any chemical peel or Laser treatment that involves exfoliation, you must avoid BHAs.

16. When should one apply a BHA?

A BHA should be applied at bedtime. Do not combine it with retinol, vitamin C and, if possible, AHAs too at the same time. It can be combined with niacinamide or hyaluronic acid.

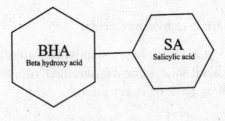

17. What are the side effects of salicylic acid?

Dryness, scaling and a burning sensation can occur with excessive or frequent use of salicylic acid.

18. I have acne-prone skin. What can I use during pregnancy since I am not allowed to use BHAs?

Azelaic acid is a dicarboxylic acid that has anti-inflammatory, antimicrobial, antioxidant and anti-comedolytic properties. It is extremely safe to use during pregnancy and can be used for mild to moderate acne, rosacea and hyperpigmentation.

POLYHYDROXY ACIDS

1. What are polyhydroxy acids and how are they useful?

Polyhydroxy acids (PHAs) are milder chemical exfoliants than AHAs and BHAs. They are thus safer to use for sensitive skin or for a rosacea-prone skin. PHAs remove the superficial dead skin layer, rendering the skin with an even tone and brighter look. The main difference between PHAs and AHAs/BHAs is that they have a higher molecular weight than AHA/BHAs, which prevents deeper penetration into the skin. They can thus be safely used for sensitive skin types. The commonly used PHAs are gluconolactone (derived from glucose), lactobionic acid (derived from lactic acid) and galactose (derived from glucose).

2. What are PHAs used for?

Up to 10 per cent PHA can be used by those with sensitive skin or rosacea to reduce the appearance of fine lines, unclog pores, cause gentle exfoliation, and obtain an even skin tone and texture.

3. Should a PHA be used in the morning or at night?

PHAs should preferably be used at night to avoid any sun-related adverse outcomes.

4. How does one use PHAs?

PHAs can be safely used three to four times a week since they are gentler than other acids, although the frequency of use depends on your individual skin type. It is generally recommended to start slow and increase as tolerated, which might mean starting twice a week then increasing use to three times a week and eventually every other day, if possible.

5. What are the side effects of PHAs?

There are usually no side effects of PHAs. Very rarely there may be redness, burning and irritation.

6. What should you not combine a PHA with?

Do not combine a PHA with retinol and vitamin C and layer it on the face together. You may use PHA on one night, Retinol on the other night and vitamin C during the day or on the third night

7. What can you combine PHAs with?

PHAs are the most versatile of the acids, which means they can be combined with plenty of other ingredients. They can be combined with retinoids when treating acne or photoaging. PHAs can be used in conjunction with hydroquinone to improve skin pigmentation and signs of aging. They can also be used after cosmetic procedures. A lot of AHAs will have a polyhydroxy acid in them. Also, this mild exfoliating agent can be combined with a non-exfoliating molecule like bakuchiol so that it removes the superficial dead skin layer and allows better penetration of the active ingredient of the serum.

RETINOIDS

1. What are retinoids?

Retinoids are vitamin A derivatives that are converted into retinoic acid for use in skincare. They are powerful anti-aging miracle molecules. Retinoid is an umbrella term for both over-the-counter retinol and prescription retinoids.

Retinoids are also available in retinaldehyde and retinol ester forms, which are comparatively mild and are available in cosmetic formulations as serums or creams.

2. What are the conditions for which retinoids can be used?

Retinoids are versatile molecules. They help reduce pigmentation and regulate sebaceous gland activity, thereby reducing acne. They also firm up the skin and stimulate collagen production, therefore helping reduce fine lines and the size of dilated pores. They cause chemo exfoliation and improve skin texture. So they can be used for acne, hyperpigmentation, antiaging and also certain skin conditions like psoriasis.

3. Can retinoids be used in the morning?

Sunlight degrades retinoids and decreases the efficacy of the product. Hence they should be used at night in order to get the maximum benefit.

4. How does one use retinoids?

Retinoids can cause irritation if used too frequently or if the formulation is too strong for your skin. Hence it should be used in very small quantities, preferably not more than a pea-sized amount. It should be used only once a day and that too at night. One should avoid using it around the nasal folds and lip corners. To begin with, it should be applied once a week and, if tolerated well, the frequency can be increased subsequently to twice or thrice a week. Always use a moisturizer after applying a retinoid and do not forget to use sunscreen in the morning.

5. At what age should one start using retinoids?

Retinoids should be avoided in children younger than ten years, but otherwise people of any age both men and women, can use retinoids. It is prescribed as a treatment for acne. If you want to use retinol serum for anti-aging, you can start at the age of thirty.

6. Who should not use retinoids?

Those who are planning to conceive should not use retinoids. Pregnant women should certainly stay away from retinoids. Those who have had an allergic reaction to retinoids should refrain from using them. If you have inflamed or excessively dry skin, refrain from using retinoids.

7. What are the side effects of retinoids?

If used in excess amounts, they can cause redness, burning, inflamed skin, a stinging sensation, itching, extreme dryness and sometimes irritation.

8. What are the various forms of retinoids available in the market and how can one decide which one to use?

Retinoic acid, Tretinoin, Isotretinoin, Tazarotene and Adapalene are the most potent forms of retinol and are usually prescribed by dermatologists. They should not be used without a dermatologist's guidance.

Retinol has become one of the most sought-after over-the-counter retinoids and is not a prescription drug. It is available as a serum and cream and is easily available at beauty stores and pharmacies.

Retinyl palmitate is the least potent OTC retinoid. It is good for those with sensitive or dry skin.

Retinaldehyde is an OTC retinoid that's stronger than retinol. If you have used a retinyl ester such as retinyl palmitate for a few months and need to step up to something stronger, this may be a good option.

9. Can retinol make my skin more sensitive and thinner?

This is a common myth. Since retinoids cause purging or sometimes dryness and the skin takes time to adapt to any retinoid, people think that retinoids make the skin sensitive. Retinoids, in fact, help build collagen and thicken the skin rather than making it thin.

10. Is it all right to use retinol with hyaluronic acid? What can you combine retinol with?

Retinoids can exacerbate dryness hence should be combined with moisturizing ingredients such as hyaluronic acid and ceramides. It is ideal to apply a moisturizer before applying a retinoid and then reapplying the moisturizer twenty minutes after so as to combat the dryness caused by retinoids. This is called the 'sandwich technique'.

BAKUCHIOL

1. What is bakuchiol and what are its benefits?

Bakuchiol is derived from the leaves and seeds of the psoralea corylifolia plant. It is a potent antioxidant, reduces skin pigmentation and has a pronounced soothing effect on the skin. Bakuchiol can also reduce the appearance of fine lines and wrinkles. It has long been used in Chinese medicine. Bakuchiol is popular as a pregnancy-safe 'natural' plant-derived retinol alternative.

2. What concentration of bakuchiol should one use?

Bakuchiol should be used in concentrations of 0.5 to 1 per cent.

3. When should one use bakuchiol?

Bakuchiol is a safe replacement for retinol, especially during pregnancy. Its action is very similar to that of retinol; it helps reduce pigmentation, fine lines and wrinkles, promotes skin regeneration and improves skin elasticity. It also helps heal the skin.

4. What is the right age to start using bakuchiol and when should one apply it?

Bakuchiol is safe for all skin types and can be used at any age. Unlike retinol, you can use bakuchiol twice a day, in the morning before a moisturizer and at night before applying your night creams and moisturizers.

5. Does bakuchiol have any side effects?

Burning, scaling and dermatitis can sometimes occur if you have sensitive skin, if your skin is very dry and flaky or if you are allergic to bakuchiol itself.

6. What should you not combine bakuchiol with?

Glycolic acid could degrade the formulation, hence should not be used with bakuchiol. Bakuchiol isn't known to negatively interact with other skincare ingredients. There are instances when you should avoid specific products when using a retinoid, such as exfoliators, toners and benzoyl peroxide as they can cause irritation. However, bakuchiol is safe to use with other products in your skincare regimen.

7. What can you combine bakuchiol with?

Bakuchiol combines well with hydrating ingredients such as squalane and PHAs.

ARBUTIN

1. What is arbutin and why is it useful?

Arbutin is a skin-lightening agent derived from leaves of different plants and trees such as bearberry, blueberry, pear and cranberry. It prevents the formation of melanin, which is responsible for pigmentation, by inhibiting the enzyme tyrosinase. It also helps lighten darks spots and blemishes and obtain an even skin tone.

2. What concentration of arbutin should one use?

Arbutin is available in two forms, alplha arbutin and beta arbutin. Alpha arbutin is better for use in your skincare regimen as it is more stable. A concentration of 2 per cent alpha arbutin is safe to use.

3. What are the conditions for which one can use alpha arbutin?

You can use alpha arbutin if you want to brighten your skin tone or if you want an even skin tone. It also helps to reduce freckles, age spots, melasma and hyperpigmentation.

4. When should I apply alpha arbutin?

Arbutin can be included both in your morning and evening skincare routine. Initially, begin using it once a day and, if tolerated well, you can apply it twice a day. However, if you use it in the morning, you must top it up with a layer of moisturizer and a sunscreen.

5. At what age can I start using alpha arbutin?

No matter what your skin type or age is, you can safely use arbutin in a concentration of 2 per cent if you have hyperpigmentation.

6. Who should not use arbutin?

Women planning conception or those who are pregnant should refrain from using arbutin because it breaks down into hydroquinone, which is unsafe during pregnancy.

7. What are the side effects of arbutin?

Sometimes redness or skin irritation can occur when using arbutin, though it is a less aggressive molecule compared to its counterparts such as hydroquinone.

8. What can you combine arbutin with?

Arbutin can be easily combined with vitamin C, liquorice extract, kojic acid, AHAs/BHAs, hyaluronic acid, glutathione and retinol. When used with other skin-lightening agents, it offers better results.

HYALURONIC ACID

1. What is hyaluronic acid and why is it useful?

Hyaluronic acid is a glycosaminoglycan (a form of glucose) and has the ability to bind with water molecules and retain moisture. It is able to hold up to a thousand times its molecular weight in water. Hyaluronic acid penetrates the skin and binds water to skin cells, hydrating all the layers of the skin. It provides moisture to the skin's natural barriers, slows down the deterioration of the lipid barrier and helps protect it. It is also biostimulatory, which means it stimulates the fibroblast cells in the skin to form new collagen. It helps in obtaining a more radiant and smooth skin.

2. What concentration of hyaluronic acid can be used?

Many skincare products contain hyaluronic acid in a concentration of 0.25 to 2.5 per cent. However, it is ideal to use it in a concentration of 1 per cent.

3. Why should one use hyaluronic acid in their skincare routine?

Hyaluronic acid alleviates dry skin, speeds up wound healing, reduces fine lines and wrinkles, and hydrates and plumps the skin. It can be used by any age group both in the morning and at night. It is especially recommended for those with mature, dry or sensitive skin.

4. When should one apply hyaluronic acid?

Hyaluronic acid serums can be used either in the morning or at night. It sits on top of the skin where it forms a layer of hydration hence can be applied at any time of the day.

5. How does one use hyaluronic acid?

Hyaluronic acid is available as a serum formulation. First, cleanse your face with a cleanser, and then apply the hyaluronic acid serum on your damp face so that it retains the moisture. Do not apply it on dry skin. Top it up with a moisturizer for better efficacy. If you are using

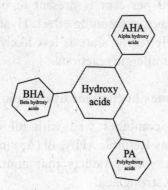

it along with a retinol or a vitamin C serum, allow the retinol serum to settle and soak into your skin for about twenty minutes and then apply the hyaluronic acid serum.

6. What age groups can use hyaluronic acid?

The aging process usually starts around the age of twenty, though visible signs start appearing when you are nearing thirty. So, it's better to start using hyaluronic acid as early as possible, especially in your early twenties, as it makes the skin more hydrated and plump and gives a youthful look to your skin.

7. Who should not use hyaluronic acid?

Since hyaluronic acid is a safe molecule, it can be used by anyone who has no history of any irritation caused by this molecule.

8. What are the side effects of hyaluronic acid?

Hyaluronic acid is naturally present in the human body. Fifty per cent of hyaluronic acid is present in skin.

The remaining 50 per cent is present in our eyes and joints, where it has a cushioning effect. Hyaluronic acid, if applied topically to the skin, is less likely to produce any side effects or allergic reactions.

9. What should one not combine hyaluronic acid with?

Hyaluronic acid combines well with all other active ingredients such as Retinol, AHA, BHA, vitamin C, etc. Avoid using HA with products that contain alcohol, fragrances or any strong acids.

10. What can you combine hyaluronic acid with?

It can be combined with products that include a retinol, vitamin C or AHAs/BHAs and niacinamide.

11. Should I apply hyaluronic acid before or after moisturizer?

Hyaluronic acid serum must be applied on damp skin before a moisturizer. However, if your skin is dry, it will pull any residual moisture from the deeper layers of the skin to hydrate the surface. In such situations, apply a light moisturizer or mist first to make the skin moist, and then apply the hyaluronic acid serum over it.

VITAMIN C

1. What is vitamin C and why is it useful?

Vitamin C is every dermatologist's favourite molecule. It is a potent antioxidant, which means it protects skin cells from damaging free radicals caused by UV exposure, pollution, stress, sugar, smoking and alcohol. It also inhibits melanin production in the skin, which helps lighten hyperpigmentation and brown spots, evens out skin tone and enhances skin radiance. It causes DNA repair and promotes collagen formation in the skin.

2. What is the ideal concentration of vitamin C that one should use?

The ideal concentration of vitamin C serum is between 10 and 20 per cent. Increasing the concentration beyond 20 per cent can cause irritation and does not offer any additional benefit. A concentration of below 8 per cent do not fetch any significant results.

3. What does vitamin C help with?

Vitamin C can reduce dark spots, blemishes, uneven skin tone, hyperpigmentation, dark circles under the eyes, sunspots and post-acne blemishes. It also helps protect the skin from UV rays, blue light and free radicles produced due to smoking and pollution. It also helps reduce fine lines and the size of open pores.

4. When should I apply vitamin C?

As vitamin C serum helps protect the skin from free radicals and UV rays, you should use it in the morning before applying sunscreen. However, L-ascorbic acid, which is the most potent form of vitamin C, is highly unstable and gets oxidized on exposure to light. Hence it is advisable to use other salts of vitamin C such as magnesium ascorbyl phosphate, ascorbyl palmitate, ethyl ascorbic acid and tetrahexyldecyl ascorbate in the morning. L-ascorbic acid formulations can be used at bedtime.

5. How should one use vitamin C?

Cleanse your face with a cleanser. Take roughly three to four drops of the vitamin C serum/cream and gently massage it all over the face including the undereye area. Wait for about five to six minutes for the serum/cream to be completely absorbed into the skin, and then you can layer it with a moisturizer and a sunscreen. Alternatively, you can use it at night before a moisturizer or a hyaluronic acid serum.

6. At what age should one start using vitamin C?

Age is no bar for vitamin C serum. It can be used by people of any age group. However, the author prescribes vitamin C to patients who are above twenty years old.

7. Who should not use vitamin C?

People with acne-prone skin should do a test patch as most vitamin C serums or cream formulations have a water in oil base, which can clog pores and result in acne. Alternatively, you can check the labels of the serums/creams and specifically use oil in water formulations to prevent acne.

8. Are there any side effects of vitamin C?

Sometimes vitamin C serums or creams can cause skin irritation, redness and burning. At times, it can cause acne to flare up if you have acne-prone skin.

9. What should one not combine vitamin C with?

Vitamin C, also known as ascorbic acid, is citric acid, which is an AHA. Layering it with other AHAs and BHAs such as glycolic, salicylic and lactic acids or retinol can destabilize the pH and render it useless. Benzoyl peroxide, a potent anti-acne ingredient, can oxidize vitamin C and make it less potent.

10. What can one combine vitamin C with?

Vitamin C works very well in combination with vitamin E and ferulic acid. You can also combine it with niacinamide and hyaluronic acid.

NIACINAMIDE

1. What is niacinamide and how is it useful?

Niacinamide is a derivative of niacin, that is, vitamin B3. It can be obtained through one's diet from meat, fish, milk, eggs and nuts. It is anti-inflammatory and helps reduce acne and post-acne blemishes. It is a potent antioxidant. It aids in skin repair and hydrates the skin by helping in the synthesis of sphingolipids, free fatty acids, cholesterol and ceramides, thus decreasing trans-epidermal water loss. Increased barrier function may mean less irritation and redness when the skin encounters environmental insults, such as detergents and soaps, hence less reddening of the skin.

The skin has pigment-forming cells called melanocytes amidst regular cells called keratinocytes. In the melanocytes lie organelles called melanosomes where the pigment melanin is synthesized and stored.

When these melanosomes are transferred to the surrounding cells, it results in hyperpigmentation or darkening of the skin. Niacinamide reduces melanosome transfer from melanocytes to the surrounding keratinocytes and thus reduces hyperpigmentation. It also increases collagen production, improves skin elasticity and reduces fine wrinkles.

2. Who can use niacinamide?

Niacinamide can be used on all skin types at any age. It is best for those with acne, rosacea or uneven skin tone. It is specifically useful for people with sensitive skin dealing with pigmentation since niacinamide doesn't have any purging effects like those of vitamin C or retinol. It is a safe vitamin, and you can combine it with any active ingredient you might be currently using in your skincare regimen. You can use it in the day or at night but start with lower concentrations of 1 to 2 per cent and always do a test patch first.

3. How should one use niacinamide?

You can use niacinamide any time in the morning or at night.

PEPTIDES

1. What are peptides?

Peptides, namely small amino acid sequences, and proteins occur naturally in the skin. They stimulate collagen production and inhibit the formation of melanin.

They are often an ingredient in many skincare products. One cosmeceutical use of peptides is as a carrier for larger molecular weight molecules to enhance penetration into the deeper layers of the skin.

2. How do peptides help in skin health?

Collagen is made of three polypeptide chains, so adding peptides can stimulate your skin to produce collagen. More collagen can lead to firmer, younger-looking skin.

3. How do peptides in skincare products work?

Peptides penetrate into the deeper layers of the skin. They are 'messengers' for the cells, as they send signals telling cells to produce collagen and elastin.

4. What are the benefits of using peptides in skincare?

Peptides help smoothen fine lines and wrinkles, decrease inflammation, improve the skin barrier, increase skin firmness and reduce pigmentation.

5. What are the different forms of peptides and what is their job in skincare?

There are three types of peptides out of which two are used in skincare:

- Signal peptides—stimulate healing, increase collagen formation and improve skin appearance.
- Carrier peptides—deliver trace elements such as copper into the skin, which helps in wound healing and enhanced collagen production.

6. What is a pentapeptide?

A pentapeptide is a carrier peptide composed of amino acids such as lysine, threonine, lysine and serine, abbreviated as KTTKS, is one of the most potent peptides found in cosmeceuticals

7. Who should use peptides?

Anyone above the age of thirty can use products containing peptides as they are excellent anti-aging ingredients. And anyone with fine lines, wrinkles, dull or sagging skin can use peptides to prevent further damage.

8. How are peptides different from other collagen-boosting ingredients?

Peptides boost collagen but also have other roles such as wound healing and reducing inflammation and hyperpigmentation.

9. How can one use peptides in one's skincare routine?

You can use serums and moisturizers containing peptides. They can be used both in the morning and at night.

10. How often should one use a peptide product?

Peptide products are safe to use twice daily. You should opt for a product that can be left on the skin, such as a cream or serum.

11. What do peptides pair well with, and what should one avoid using them with?

Peptides work well with ingredients such as vitamin C, niacinamide, antioxidants and hyaluronic acid. Using a peptide with an AHA will reduce the efficacy of the peptides.

OTHER RELATED QUESTIONS

1. There is a lot of talk about centella asiatica. How good is it for skin?

Centella asiatica, commonly known as mandukparni, Indian pennywort or gotu kola, has been used as a medicine in the Ayurvedic tradition of India for thousands of years. The most important constituents isolated from C. asiatica are triterpenoid saponins, which increase the percentage of collagen and a protein called fibronectin in the skin. They help in wound healing and scar management and are present in most creams for stretch marks. They are also present in anti-aging creams and serums as they boost collagen and moisturize the skin.

2. Is rose hip oil worth the hype?

Rose hips, the red, fleshy berries of the dog rose (Rosa canina), are particularly rich in vitamin C, carotenoids, polyphenols and various flavonoids that have potent antioxidant activity. The seeds contained within the rose hips have been shown to comprise high amounts of polyunsaturated fatty acids, known to have anti-inflammatory properties. Rose hip oil is thus known to hydrate the skin, reduce fine lines and help in skin firmness. It does not usually have any side effects.

3. What are the benefits of marine collagen?

Marine collagen peptides are obtained from fish or algae. They have antioxidant and anti-inflammatory properties. They are available in the form of oral supplements, and topical serums and creams. They also help in collagen synthesis and wound healing. Astaxanthin is one such potent marine collagen that has shown anti-aging benefits when taken as capsules and applied in the form of creams. The ability of marine collagen to promote skin re-epithelization and collagen regeneration makes it better than land animal collagen. Besides, collagen from algae can also be used by vegetarians.

RAPID FIRE

1. What serum can one use if one has sensitive skin?

Polyhydroxy acids are safe for sensitive skin, however, please consult a dermatologist before you use any serums.

2. What serum can one use if one has combination skin?

Lactic acid, hyaluronic acid, vitamin C and niacinamide can be used for combination skin.

L. Phetcharat, K. Wongsuphasawat, K. Winther. The Effectiveness of a Standardized Rose Hip Powder, Containing Seeds and Shells of Rosa Canina, on Cell Longevity, Skin Wrinkles, Moisture, and Elasticity. *Clinical Interventions in Aging*. 2015; 10: 1849–1856. Published 19 November 2015. doi:10.2147/CIA.S90092

S. Geahchan, P. Baharlouei, A. Rahman. Marine Collagen: A Promising Biomaterial for Wound Healing, Skin Anti-Aging, and Bone Regeneration. *Marine Drugs*. 2022; 20 (1): 61. Published January 10 2022. doi:10.3390/md20010061

3. Can I use snail mucin on my face every day? I am 30 years old and have dry skin.

Snail mucin is said to contain allantoin, hyaluronic acid and glycolic acid. It has antioxidant properties. You may use it daily if you have no allergic reaction to it. Do a test patch and see. Unfortunately, there isn't enough scientific evidence proving its benefits yet.

4. Can I use peptides with retinol?

Yes, you can safely use peptides with retinol.

5. Is it necessary to store vitamin C serum in the refrigerator?

No. However, L ascorbic acid does get oxidized when exposed to light. Hence always store it in a cool dark place.

6. Which is the best retinoid to use if I am a first-time user?

Retinyl esters are the least potent and mildest form of retinoids. So, they are the safest for beginners.

7. What should you not combine a retinoid with?

Retinols should not be combined with vitamin C, benzoyl peroxide and AHAs/BHAs together at the same time as they can cause irritation.

8. Can hyaluronic acid make the skin dry?

If hyaluronic acid is applied on dry skin and if the environment is dry too, it sucks moisture from the deeper skin layers, making the skin even more dry. Second, some formulations contain large molecules of HA which may not be able to penetrate the skin adequately.

8

Serums

'A serum is like a bindi used in the centre of the forehead by Hindus. It comes in various forms for various skin needs.'

—Jaishree Sharad

A serum is a step ahead of using a moisturizer and sunscreen. A serum has a specific function and can be added in one's skincare routine according to one's skin requirement. For example, hyperpigmented skin would need niacinamide, dehydrated skin would need hyaluronic acid, aging skin would need retinoids and so on. Lets dig into the world of serums.

1. What are serums? How are they different from creams and lotions?

Serums are liquids containing highly concentrated active ingredients that can be used for specific skin conditions.

They are usually water-based although a few serums may be oil-based. The particle size of a serum is much smaller than that of a cream or a gel. Serums do not contain heavy occlusive ingredients such as petrolatum, mineral oil, beeswax, etc. Hence they can penetrate the skin more easily.

2. Why should serums be used?

Serums are easier to use and contain a higher concentration of ingredients. Those with problematic skin such as acne, hyperpigmentation, dilated pores or fine lines should incorporate serums in their skincare routine. Also, if you do not prefer thick greasy products and you want something lightweight, you may opt for serums. As you age, your skin will need a serum in addition to a moisturizer and sunscreen.

3. Who should not be using serums?

People with oily skin or acne-prone skin should avoid an oil-based vitamin C serum. If you have very sensitive skin or conditions such as eczema and rosacea, which tend to weaken the skin barrier, you should avoid serums containing chemical exfoliants such as AHA and BHA as they can penetrate the skin easily and cause more irritation.

4. Is a serum the same as an essence?

A serum is more concentrated and has a thicker consistency as compared to an essence. An essence is watery and doesn't contain a very high concentration of active ingredients as compared to serums. An essence cannot be used as a single skincare product while a serum can be used alone.

5. When should a serum be applied in the skincare routine?

A serum should be applied immediately after cleansing the face, before a moisturizer and sunscreen. Similarly, at bedtime, after removing make-up and cleansing the face, a serum should be applied on the entire face followed by either the moisturizer or the targeted cream or anti-aging cream. If you apply a cream before a serum, the cream will lock the skin and not allow the serum to penetrate the skin. Hence always use a serum before a cream, sunscreen or oil.

6. What quantity of serum should be applied on the face and how should one apply it?

Since a serum is very concentrated, a little goes a long way. Three to five drops are enough for the entire face and neck. Just dot the entire face with the serum and gently massage it into the skin till it is completely absorbed. Too much of anything can harm the skin, so do not use large amounts of the serum.

7. I have dry skin. Which serum should I use?

If you have dry skin, you can use hyaluronic acid-based serums. Hyaluronic acid is a normal ingredient in the skin, in the joints, even in the eyes and is a hydrating agent. One-fourth of a teaspoon of HA can absorb half a gallon of water and keep the skin hydrated. Another serum for dry skin is a niacinamide-based serum. Niacinamide is vitamin B3. It helps in the formation of ceramides, which are the building blocks in the skin. Niacinamide is also a potent anti-inflammatory and an antioxidant. Hence it is not only hydrating but it also protects the skin from free radical scavengers. Avoid serums containing AHA, BHA or retinol in them without a dermatologist's recommendation.

8. I often develop acne on my face. Should I be using a serum at all? If yes, which one?

If you have acne-prone or oily skin, you can use a serum containing beta hydroxy acid such as salicylic acid. Beta hydroxy acid is lipid-soluble so it will penetrate the skin through the oil ducts and enter the oil glands. It will dissolve the sebum or the oil in the skin and help unclog pores, and it also helps reduce oiliness. However, beta hydroxy acid is not safe for use during pregnancy. You may also use an alpha hydroxy acid such as glycolic acid or mandelic acid. Alpha hydroxy acids help in exfoliating dead skin, making the skin texture smoother, and also help in making the skin less oily. You could use a retinol-based serum twice a week if you have oily or acne-prone skin. Use a very small amount at bedtime, and make sure you always moisturize and use a sunscreen during the day when you are applying retinol on your skin. Retinol helps reduce acne and oiliness, and it helps exfoliate the skin; however, it is not safe to use during pregnancy. Do not use retinol along with an AHA or a BHA on the same day.

9. Please suggest a serum which can reduce fine lines on the face.

If you have fine lines, you could use hyaluronic acid to plump the skin. You could also use alpha hydroxy acids such as glycolic acid or retinol or a vitamin C serum, all of which stimulate the collagen and elastin fibres and help reduce fine lines.

10. Will a serum reduce my enlarged pores?

Serums will help in reducing pores by only about 30 to 40 per cent. It also depends on the severity of the damage. Severely dilated pores will require interventions such as microneedling, radio frequency microneedling, fractional Lasers or platelet-rich plasma treatment.

If you have dilated pores with oily skin, alternate between a BHA serum, which will unclog the pores, and an AHA-based serum, which will tighten the pores. If you have dilated pores with mature aging skin or normal-to-dry skin, you should use a retinol, vitamin C or AHA-based serum to stimulate collagen and tighten the pores.

11. My face is darker in some areas and lighter in others. What serum should I use?

If you have hyperpigmentation or uneven skin tone, opt for a vitamin C or niacinamide-based serum. Another ingredient that can help is kojic acid. Kojic acid is obtained from a mushroom extract. It inhibits the enzyme tyrosinase. Tyrosinase helps in the production of the pigment melanin. Tranexamic acid serums are also beneficial for hyperpigmentation. You can alternate any of these with an AHA or retinol-based serum for better results.

12. What serum should be used under the eyes?

If you have hyperpigmentation or dark circles, you can use a serum that contains ingredients such as vitamin C, alpha arbutin, kojic acid, liquorice or green tea. If you have puffiness under the eyes, use a serum with vitamin K, or caffeine or green tea in it. If you have fine lines and wrinkles under eyes, use a retinol-, peptide- or resveratrol-based serum.

13. Can I skip a moisturizer if I use a hyaluronic acid-based serum?

If you have oily or acne-prone skin, you can skip the moisturizer, but make sure you apply the HA serum on slightly damp skin to lock the moisture in the skin. But if you have dry skin, a moisturizer is a must over a hyaluronic acid-based serum, else the hyaluronic acid may absorb water from the deeper layers of your skin and cause more dryness.

14. I had an acne outbreak after using a vitamin C-based serum. Isn't it necessary to use a vitamin C-based serum in your twenties?

Not at all. If your skin cannot tolerate something, it tells you that it doesn't need it. Vitamin C is a great active ingredient but not a necessity, as is the case with other active ingredients. The only absolute skin necessity is a sunscreen.

15. What are antioxidant serums?

Free radicals are toxins in the body that can damage the DNA, proteins and lipids in the skin and cause cell damage.

Our body is exposed to free radicals through pollution, soot, smoke, chemicals, nicotine, stress, hormones, digestive by-products and even certain medicines. These free radicals are scavenged by antioxidants. Antioxidants can be obtained through food or supplements.

Vitamins C and E, ferulic acid, some minerals such as selenium and chromium, flavonoids found in herbal teas, berries and red wine are powerful antioxidants. Blackberries, cranberries, blueberries, beans, artichokes, pecans, walnuts and hazelnuts are foods thought to be the richest in antioxidants.

Antioxidants are also available in anti-aging serums containing vitamin C, resveratrol, alpha lipoic acid, vitamin E, ferulic acid, retinol and coffee berry.

16. What is skin purging? Does it occur with all ingredients?

When you use ingredients like retinol, AHA or BHA, there is microexfoliation of the skin and a temporary flare up of acne in the form of papules or pustules (tiny whiteheads with or without pus). This is more common in people with acne prone or oily skin. This effect lasts only for four to six weeks, after which the skin begins to get normal. Hence one should not stop using the retinol or AHA or BHA if they see a flare up of acne.

However, if you develop acne after using a vitamin C or niacinamide or hyaluronic acid, that is a reaction and not purging.

FACE MASKS

1. I have oily skin. Should I be using a clay mask, charcoal mask or a sheet mask?

A charcoal mask will suit you best. Charcoal has the property of de-greasing the skin and unclogging pores. It will reduce the oil and also help in getting rid of superficial blackheads. A clay mask can also be used if you have oily skin, but do not use it too often as it tends to dry out the skin. Sheet masks may be used for a glow, but they do not reduce oil.

2. Are clay masks better or sheet masks?

It depends on the skin type and skin concern. If you have dry, dehydrated skin, you should opt for sheet masks. If you have oily or acne-prone skin, clay masks are better. If you have normal skin, you can use either. If you have sensitive skin, you can use sheet masks with mild ingredients such as hyaluronic acid.

3. Should I wash my face before applying a sheet mask?

Whether you apply a sheet mask, clay mask or charcoal mask, it is very important to remove all make-up and cleanse the face. Otherwise you will be trapping make-up, dust, dirt, grime, sebum, sweat salts and dead skin beneath the mask, resulting in clogged pores and even acne.

4. Do I have to dry my skin completely before applying a face mask?

Wash your face with warm water and apply the mask immediately. The ingredients in the mask penetrate better when the face is warm and slightly damp.

5. For how long should I leave the mask on my face?

If your face mask contains retinol, AHA, BHA or, if you are using clay/charcoal masks, you should not leave them on for too long as they will dry out the skin. Leaving them on for fifteen to twenty minutes should be enough. Other masks can be left on for longer periods; however, read the instructions on the package and follow them strictly.

6. Can you elaborate on which ingredients to look for in masks?

The ingredients will depend on your skin type and the reason why you require a mask.

If you have acne, opt for clay masks, charcoal masks or masks with AHA, BHA or sulphur, which will help reduce oiliness, blackheads and whiteheads, and unclog pores. If you have dull or tanned skin, you can use sheet masks containing kojic acid, liquorice, vitamin C, coffee berry, soy, etc., to brighten the skin. Fruit enzyme masks such as papaya or pumpkin work best for dull skin. Hyaluronic acid and glycerine face masks are great for hydration.

RAPID FIRE

1. Please suggest a serum for oily skin.

All the serums mentioned for acne-prone skin can be used for oily skin.

2. What is a good anti-aging serum?

Serums containing retinol, resveratrol, argireline and peptides are good anti-aging serums.

3. I have very sensitive skin. What serum can I use for radiant skin?

Serums containing polyhydroxy acid or niacinamide may be better for you. But do try a test patch.

4. If AHA causes purging, what should I do?

Just use a moisturizer and continue to use the AHA. Purging is a normal skin reaction and will stop in four to six weeks.

5. Which serum should I use for glowing skin?

Serums with AHA, retinol, niacinamide or vitamin C can all be used.

6. Can I use a salicylic acid-based serum daily?

If you have very oily or acne-prone skin with clogged pores, you may use SA daily unless your skin feels dry or flaky. If you have normal, dry or sensitive skin, it is better to use it on alternate nights or twice a week depending on the skin dryness.

7. If I want to use retinol, hyaluronic acid and a vitamin C serum, how do I layer these products?

It is best not to layer vitamin C with retinol. Use vitamin C in the morning and apply hyaluronic acid at night followed by retinol.

8. Vitamin C makes my skin brownish when I apply it. What should I do?

Your vitamin C has oxidized. You need to discard it and buy a new bottle. Always store vitamin C in a cool, dark place.

9. What serums are safe to use during pregnancy?

Serums based on niacinamide, hyaluronic acid, vitamin C and AHAs can be used during pregnancy.

10. Can I use a serum if I have rosacea ?

Yes, a polyhydroxy acid or niacinamide serum will help.

11. Can I use a lactic acid serum in the morning and a retinol cream at night? I have oily skin.

It is better to use them on alternate nights. The skin doesn't need too much chemo exfoliation. Overexfoliation may damage the barrier protective layer of the skin.

12. What is skin cycling?

When you use retinol one night, AHA or BHA the next night and a moisturizer or HA for the remaining two consecutive nights, allowing the skin to heal from the exfoliating effects of retinol or AHA and BHA, it is called skin cycling. It is better than using all the serums daily.

9

Layering of Skincare Products

'Your skin has a memory. In ten, twenty, thirty years from now, your skin will show the results of how it was treated today. So treat it kindly and with respect.'

—Violet Grey

Just as you layer your clothes or follow a sequence for anything for the end result to be good, you need to layer your skincare products right. More importantly, you want the products to penetrate the skin properly. You may have the best products but you if you don't layer them correctly, their efficacy would be compromised. So whether you layer three products or ten, the steps should be in the right order.

1. What is layering skincare?

Layering is applying skincare products in a particular order.

2. Is layering of products good for the skin?

Appropriate application of the right products in the right order according to your skin's needs is the basis of layering. Using too many products all the time can damage your skin.

3. How does one layer skincare products?

Use products with the thinnest texture first, moving on to products with thicker texture and the thickest texture at the end. Apply water-based products before oil-based ones. Give your products one to two minutes to get absorbed, before moving on to the next step. Sunscreen is the only product which needs fifteen minutes of absorption time before you apply make-up over it.

So, after cleansing your face, use a serum followed by a moisturizer and then the sunscreen. If you are applying make-up, it should be applied over the sunscreen. At bedtime, cleanse, apply a serum, then apply the targeted cream if you need to and top it up with a moisturizer. If you use a mask, it should be applied over the moisturizer. A mask should be the last step in your bedtime skincare ritual.

4. What goes first, moisturizer or vitamin C?

Vitamin C should be applied before the moisturizer. Any product with a thin consistency should be applied first.

Moisturizer, being thicker, is applied later. Apply a few drops of vitamin C, wait for five minutes and then apply a moisturizer.

5. How should I layer my products in the day and at night?

Daycare routine

Always begin with a cleanser followed by a toner or essence and serum. However, the usage of a toner and serum is completely optional. Then apply a moisturizer for the face and neck and on top of it apply a sunscreen. Make sure that the sunscreen is always the topmost layer. Then moisturize your arms, hands, legs and feet and again apply sunscreen on all the exposed body parts.

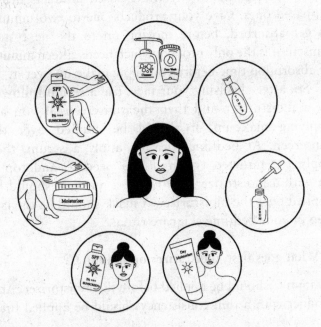

Nightcare routine

Begin with the removal of your make-up if you are wearing any, using a make-up remover or cleansing lotion. Then, wash your face using a facewash that suits your skin type to cleanse your face. Following this, gently dab an under-eye serum on the skin under the eyes. Be careful not to rub the product in as skin under the eyes is very thin. Then apply a face serum that is suitable for your skin type and skin condition. Depending on your need, you can even apply a targeted cream for aging, acne, pigmentation, pores, etc., but these creams can be skipped, especially if you are under forty years old. Next, moisturize your face and neck with a suitable moisturizer. You may wrap it up with a mask over the moisturizer.

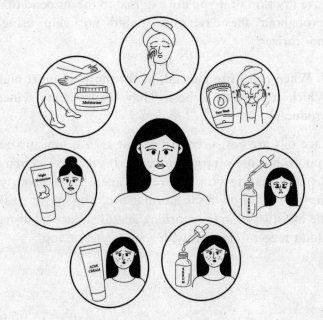

Do not forget to apply a moisturizer on other parts of your body such as hands, legs and feet.

6. Are toners good or bad to use?

Toners are not an essential part of skincare. However, they are used to remove all traces of oil, make-up and dirt from the skin. Non-alcohol-based toners are available. So, if you want to use a toner, it should be used right after cleansing, before using a serum.

7. Can I skip using a moisturizer if I use a serum and sunscreen ?

If you have oily skin and you are using a niacinamide-based serum, you can skip using a moisturizer. If you have dry skin or if you are exposed to the air conditioner throughout the day, you should not skip using a moisturizer.

8. When can I use face oil, in the morning or at night? Which step would it be if I have to layer my skincare products?

Face oils are best used at bedtime over a moisturizer if you do not use a targeted cream. If you have extremely dry and mature skin (above the age of forty-five), you may use a face oil in the morning too. You may even skip the moisturizer in the morning and use a face oil instead. Don't forget to layer it with a sunscreen on top.

9. I am in my mid-forties and have oily skin. Can I use a face mask? If yes, what type and when can I use it in my skincare?

Face masks are available as either gels or creams. It is the last layer of the skincare routine and can be left overnight. You should opt for gel-based masks which contain active ingredients such as niacinamide, collagen, retinol or peptides.

10. Should one apply retinol as the first layer or the last layer in the night time skincare routine?

Retinol should be used as the last layer over a moisturizer at bedtime.

If one experiences dryness after applying retinol, or during winter, it can be applied using the sandwich technique. After applying moisturizer, apply retinol and follow it with another layer of moisturizer.

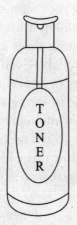

11. If I want to use niacinamide and vitamin C serum, how do I layer it?

It is better to use niacinamide serum in the morning and vitamin C serum at bedtime or vice versa instead of layering them one on top of the other. However, if you still want to use both serums together, apply the lighter and thinner one first.

12. Is glass skin achievable?

Glass skin, a term made popular by Korean beauties, is not a miracle. Glass skin refers to crystal-clear, blemish free, translucent and radiant skin that looks like a piece of clear glass. One cannot achieve glass skin overnight. It takes months of following a regular skincare regime to make your skin look like glass. However, it is not impossible to achieve.

Some of the steps you can follow are, at bedtime, remove all make-up from your face with a hydrating make-up remover or baby oil. Cleanse your face with a facewash that suits your skin type and then apply a hydrating serum containing hyaluronic acid or vitamin C and vitamin E. Hydrating sheet masks (there are plenty of Korean brands available) can also be used instead of serums. The serum or sheet mask is left overnight, allowing the skin to soak in the solution and enhancing complete absorption of the ingredients into the skin. In the morning, cleanse your face with plain water or a soap-free cleanser. Follow this with a moisturizer suitable for your skin type. Top it with a sunscreen that protects your skin from UVA and UVB rays. Make sure you avoid alcohol, nicotine and sugar, and sleep for at least six hours daily. Repeat this simple regime every single day for at least six months and you will see the transformation in the texture and tone of your skin. The results will be gratifying, but the key is to maintain it by following these steps routinely.

13. Can you provide an age-wise skincare routine as I have a teenager in my house and a twenty-six-year-old. I myself am forty-eight and my husband is fifty-eight.

That's an all-in-one question. Teenagers should keep it simple and use a cleanser, moisturizer and sunscreen in the morning and a cleanser and moisturizer at bedtime. If they have acne, they can add an anti-acne cream as prescribed by their dermatologist.

In your twenties, you can add vitamin C in the morning, before you moisturize. If you have blemishes, add lactic or glycolic acid serum at bedtime before your night moisturizer. However, if you have acne-prone skin, use niacinamide serum in the morning and a salicylic acid serum at bedtime before applying moisturizer.

In your thirties, you can add a retinol or peptide at night, and if the skin is dry, you can also add hyaluronic acid.

In your forties and above, you may need a serum containing vitamin C or AHA or BHA or retinol or peptides or hyaluronic acid depending on your skin type and concern. So, you need to consult a dermatologist before buying any skincare products.

A quick guide to layering of skincare products

Daycare
Step 1 – Cleanser
Step 2 – Toner or essence or mist (optional)
Step 3 – Serum (optional) Step 4 – Eye cream or serum (optional) Step 5 – Light face oil (optional)
Step 6 – Moisturizer for face and neck
Step 7 – Heavy Face oil (optional, if skin very dry) Step 8 – Sunscreen
Step 9 – Moisturizer for arms, hands, legs and feet
Step 10 – Sunscreen for exposed body parts
Nightcare
Step 1 – Remove make-up
Step 2 – Cleanse Step 3 – Exfoliate (optional, don't do it daily) Step 4 – Toner or mist (optional)
Step 5 – Under-eye serum
Step 4 – Targeted serum
Step 5 – Targeted creams
Step 6 – Moisturizer for face and neck
Step 7 – Moisturizer for hands, legs and feet

10

Neck Skincare

'We all look good for our age. Except for our necks.'
—Nora Ephron

The skin over the neck is thin and lacks sebaceous glands. Since the dermis is thinner, the collagen and elastin fibers are less as compared to the face. Hence the neck is more prone to wrinkles and fine lines. The neck has a sheet of muscle called the platysma which runs in bands from the clavicle to the mouth.

When one strains the neck at the gym by lifting heavy weights regularly, there is exertion on the platysma which eventually forms vertical bands on the neck. Similarly, if you constantly look down at your phone or laptop, the horizontal lines on your neck become prominent over time.

The neck needs as much attention as your face. Do not neglect it.

1. Why does the neck look older in some people who have youthful faces?

People tend to neglect the neck when it comes to skincare. They spend a great deal of time and attention improving the skin of the face because it is a mindset. They do not realize that the neck ages too. They see only the face, not realizing that the neck skin is a continuation of the face skin. So, if you apply creams and undergo treatments for the face so that your face looks youthful, your neck will be an age giveaway and will also age faster.

2. How different is the skin on the neck from the skin on the face?

The skin on the neck is a bit thinner than that on the face as the dermis on the neck is thinner as compared to that on the face. There are fewer skin appendages such as sweat or oil glands or hair present in the neck skin.

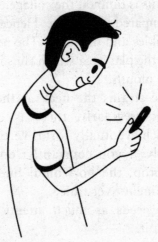

Neck skin is much drier and more prone to wrinkling. There is very little fat in the neck, which is why the skin tends to sag sooner.

3. Why does one develop skin folds or bands on the neck, and what should one do to prevent them?

Fine lines, wrinkles, sagging of skin, horizontal neck bands, turkey legs or vertical neck bands are a result of glycation, stress, bad lifestyle, zero skincare for the neck and of course, normal, intrinsic aging.

To prevent premature aging of the neck, whatever serum, moisturizer, sunscreen and night cream you apply on the face should be applied on the neck as well.

4. What can I do for vertical bands on my neck? I am thirty-eight years old and I hate these bands.

Vertical bands on the neck occur due to the platysma muscle, which lies in the neck like a sheet. Overactivity of the muscle while clenching your teeth or lifting weights or just the process of aging can result in these

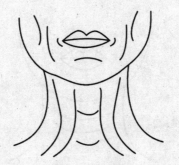

neck bands. Tiny doses of botulinum toxin injections all along the neck bands not only improve them, they also improve the jawline definition and neck firmness. The treatment is safe and approved by the US Food and Drug Administration (FDA), but should be performed only by a well-trained, qualified dermatologist or plastic surgeon. The effect of the injection lasts for four to five months after which one needs to repeat the injections. The skin does not lose its elasticity with repeated injections. So, please consult a dermatologist and get botulinum toxin injections done before these bands become worse.

5. What treatments help prevent neck aging? At what age can one start these preventative treatments?

Apart from routine skincare, one can opt for preventative anti-aging treatments for the neck at the age of thirty or above. Microneedling, platelet-rich plasma therapy, chemical peels and skin booster injections are safe anti-aging treatments that prevent premature aging of the neck.

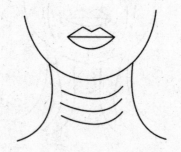

6. My neck seems to have darkened and thickened over time. How can this be corrected?

Some people can develop a thick, dark, velvety band or patch on the neck, which is mistaken for dirt. This is a condition called acanthosis nigricans. It can occur due to insulin resistance, diabetes, Cushing's disease, polycystic ovarian syndrome, hypothyroidism, raised prolactin levels, obesity or could also be caused by oral contraceptive pills or oral steroids. Please consult a dermatologist to identify the cause. If you are obese or your BMI is more than twenty-five, it is extremely important to lose weight and bring the BMI to twenty-five or less.

Regular exercise and a healthy diet are equally important. You must stop having sugar in any form. Cane sugar, jaggery, organic sugar, coconut sugar, dates and honey should be completely stopped. Your physician may also prescribe metformin tablets for insulin resistance. Creams containing lactic acid and urea can help reduce the dark colour. Sometimes even chemical peels are done to get rid of the hyperpigmentation that persists after weight loss.

7. Besides acanthosis nigricans, what other diseases can affect the neck?

Deficiency of folic acid or vitamin B12, intertrigo (inflammation in the folds of the skin) due to sweat and friction, fungal infections like tinea corporis and tinea versicolor, skin tags and warts can also result in darkening of the neck. The other skin disorders that can affect the neck are eczema, psoriasis, vitiligo, ashy dermatosis, lichen planus pigmentosus.

8. Of late, people are talking of the 'tech neck'—fine lines and wrinkles that appear on the neck due to constantly looking down at computer screens. What is your take on this?

Tech neck refers to horizontal lines on the neck due to looking down at mobile phones, laptops or computers for extended periods of time. The constant pull of muscles due to the neck posture causes these dynamic lines on the skin, which become static horizontal creases with time. To prevent tech neck, improve your posture by doing neck exercises and yoga. Applying sunscreen on the neck daily, and using anti-aging and hydrating neck creams that contain hyaluronic acid, glycerine, ceramides, N acetal glucosamine for hydration, alpha and beta hydroxy acids for exfoliation and retinol for anti-aging daily can also help prevent tech neck. The horizontal lines that are already formed will not disappear with creams. To remove them, one may need radio frequency or ultrasound skin tightening, skin booster injections, or low G prime hyaluronic acid filler injections.

9. A lot of brands have come out with specialized neck creams. What is your take on these? Are these necessary/ effective?

Skincare involves care for all body parts and not just the face. Hence care for the neck skin is also important. Neck creams for lifting and anti-aging purposes may contain hyaluronic acid, glycerine, ceramides, N acetal glucosamine for hydration, alpha hydroxy acid, retinol, peptides, resveratrol, etc. These can be used as night creams in your skincare ritual.

However, whatever products you use for the face can be used on the neck as well without having to buy specific neck creams.

10. What are the specialized treatments that target the skin on the neck?

Various treatments that are done for the neck are:

- Silk peel: Also known as dermal infusion or diamond glow, this is a three-in-one technique that includes exfoliation, unclogging of pores and infusion of various serums such as vitamin C, skin-brightening serum or hyaluronic acid. This treatment hydrates, nourishes and gives a glow to the skin. It also helps in lymphatic drainage of the neck.
- Non-surgical radio frequency skin-tightening treatments such as Endymed, Thermage and Exilis. These are FDA-approved devices that use radio frequency energy to tighten the skin. The procedure is painless and safe. It is done once a week for six weeks and repeated after a year. Results are seen three months after the first session.
- High intensity microfocused ultrasound (HIFU) or Ultherapy: This is an FDA-approved non-invasive device that uses high intensity microfocused ultrasound to improve wrinkles and skin laxity

on the neck. It works by using ultrasound waves for collagen remodelling. Usually, two sessions spaced three months apart are required. The results are evident after three months of the first session. The results last for a year or even up to a year and a half.

- Skin boosters: These are hyaluronic acid shots that are given to stimulate collagen production. Profhilo, Juvederm Volite, Restylane Vital and Belotero Revive are various brands of skin boosters that can be taken by anyone above the age of twenty-eight. They are neither botox nor fillers. They are literally moisturizers being injected into your skin to hydrate the skin, boost collagen and make the neck look firmer.

- Microneedling radio frequency: It involves a combination of heat energy using radio frequency and microneedling and is a good option to stimulate collagen and firm the skin. It is a safe lunchtime, in-clinic procedure and can even be done as early as the age of twenty-five. It is usually done once a month for four to six sessions.

- Platelet-rich plasma: Approximately 8 to 10 ml of your blood is collected in a specific kit and centrifuged to separate the platelet-rich plasma from the rest of the blood cells. This platelet-rich plasma concentrate is rich in various growth factors that stimulate the collagen in the skin and help in firming the neck skin. For best results, one should undergo three to four sessions at a month's interval.

- Botox: This is used to treat vertical neck bands also known as turkey legs. However, this treatment is not effective in older people who have loose skin folds.
- Microbotox is nothing but super diluted botulinum toxin, which is injected all over the neck to tighten the neck and reduce horizontal neck lines.
- Fillers: Low G prime fillers are injected into the horizontal lines on the neck to reduce them. The results last for about a year.
- Thread lifts: Cog threads, PDO threads, Silhouette threads and Aptos threads are inserted into the neck to tighten the skin. The results last for six months to a year depending on the type of thread used and the number of threads inserted.

RAPID FIRE

1. Can exercise make my vertical neck bands prominent?

Make a concious effort not to strain your neck or clench your teeth while exercising and you can avoid neck bands.

2. I have thick, dark bands on my neck for three years. Is it due to accumulation of dirt?

No, please get your hormones checked for insulin resistance, diabetes, PCOS or hypothyroidism. You may either be suffering from one of them or may be obese.

3. If I take Botox injections on my neck for my prominent neck bands, will my neck become stiff ?

Not at all. Make sure you choose a qualified injector.

4. I am seventy years old and have very loose, sagging skin on my neck. Is there a non-surgical treatment I can opt for?

Loose skin resulting in sagging and folds at any age above sixty may not respond to non-surgical modalities of treatment. The best option for you would be a neck lift surgery.

5. Is it safe to do Laser radiofrequency or HIFU treatments on the neck?

As long as your physician or therapist avoids the region of the thyroid over the neck, all of the above treatments are very safe.

11

Hand and Foot Care

'Don't judge me by the wrinkles on my hands. They
have toiled relentlessly and are oblivious of comfort.'
—Dr Jaishree Sharad

Hands face the wrath of all the work you do throughout
the day. Besides, they get exposed to dirt, pollution,
detergents, soaps and these days even sanitizers ever so
frequently in the day. In fact, the skin on the hands is the
first to show signs of aging.

Our feet need extra attention. They bear the weight of
the entire body after all. Besides, eczema, cuts and cracks
can occur at any age. Be kind to your hands and feet.
Take care of them every day.

1. What are the basic steps in hand care?

Wash your hands with normal, lukewarm or cold water.
Avoid using hot water to wash your hands as this will

zap moisture from your skin. Use a gentle, soap-free handwash. Harsh, lather-forming soaps can alter the pH of your skin making it more alkaline and dry. After every handwash, dab your skin gently and apply a moisturizer over slightly damp skin for better moisturization. Do not forget to use a sunscreen on your hands if you want to protect your hands from premature aging. At bedtime, wash your hands again and apply a thick moisturizer or even coconut or almond oil on slightly damp hands. This will trap the moisture in your skin and keep your skin hydrated. If possible, wear mittens over the moisturized hands before sleeping. Mittens will help retain the moisturizer for a longer period of time and thus help in the repair of your skin.

2. I sanitize my hands very often. Should I be taking any extra care for my hands?

Alcohol-based sanitizers can damage the barrier layer of your skin and dehydrate your skin. Washing too often or repetitive sanitizing can cause peeling of the skin or even cuts. One must reapply a fragrance-free moisturizer after every handwash and every time you sanitize your hands. Keep a hand moisturizer with you at all times. Regular moisturizing will repair your skin and keep your hands soft and supple. During the day, you can use a lighter moisturizer that does not make your hands greasy. Look for emollients such as aloe vera, lanolin, squalene, fatty acids or ceramides. Humectant ingredients such as hyaluronic acid, panthenol, urea or sorbitol can also be used during the day as they absorb water from the environment and retain it in the skin.

3. Can I use the same moisturizer for my hands in the day and night?

Yes, you may use the same moisturizer all day long. However, it is better to use a thicker and more occlusive moisturizer at bedtime. It is inconvenient to use thick moisturizers during the day as they are sticky and greasy and will be a hindrance while you work with your hands. Also, moisturizers containing occlusives and emollients will hydrate and repair your skin at night. It is better to look for ingredients such as oils, wax, petrolatum, shea butter, mango butter, cocoa butter, ceramides, etc. in your night moisturizer.

4. Should I take special precautions for my hands while doing my household chores?

Whether it is dishwashing or washing clothes or even cooking or cutting vegetables and fruit, hands bear the brunt of harsh soaps, detergents and acids from the vegetables and fruit. These can not only dry out your skin but also damage the protective barrier layer of the skin, resulting in cuts, irritant contact dermatitis, eczemas and hand allergies. Wear gloves while washing clothes or doing the dishes or mopping to prevent prolonged contact of harsh soaps with the skin. It may be wise to do all the washing together at one time instead of repeatedly washing fewer dishes throughout the day. Use a scoop to add the soap or detergent to the clothes in the washing machine. You may also opt for a dishwasher in case of severe hand eczema. Use a good hand moisturizer after washing clothes or dishes or mopping the floor. Before cooking or cutting vegetables or fruit, it may be wise to apply cooking oil or ghee to your hands. Oil is an occlusive and will form a protective layer on your skin so that the acids from the fruit and vegetables do not damage your skin.

5. What are some of the enemies of our skin?

A dry environment, low humidity, heaters, air conditioners, harsh bathing soaps and handwashes, sanitizers, disinfectants, alcohol-based hand products, exposure to grease, dirt, acids, chalk, dust, some topical or oral medicines like higher concentrations of retinol or peeling agents, frequent obsessive handwashing, frequent manicures, smoking, etc. can all affect our skin adversely.

6. I have a lot of wrinkles on my hands and they make me look very old. What can I do about it?

Frequent use of detergents, disinfectants, improper hand care, not using a moisturizer or sunscreen on your hands from as early as the age of sixteen, cold climates, excessive exposure to air conditioners or room heaters and smoking can all cause premature aging of the hands. First of all, follow the basic tips for hand care mentioned above. Never forget to use a moisturizer and sunscreen. You may use a chemical exfoliant such as an AHA or retinol twice a week. Alpha hydroxy acid peels such as glycolic acid, lactic acid or mandelic acid peels once a month can also help in mild exfoliation and an improvement in mild fine lines on the hand. At the clinic, microneedling with Dermapen is another easy and safe treatment for fine lines on the hands. Slightly more severe lines may need fractional Laser resurfacing. Dry and wrinkled hands can be treated with skin booster injections. These injections contain hyaluronic acid, which not only hydrates the skin and makes the hands look supple and soft, it also stimulates collagen and elastin fibres, making the skin firm and wrinkle-free. Severe hollowing, folds and wrinkles on the hand would benefit from filler injections. Hyaluronic acid fillers (Juvederm, Restylane, Belotero), calcium hydroxylapatite fillers (Radiesse) and poly L lactic acid fillers (Sculptra) are great for aging hands. The effect lasts for about one to one-and-a-half years and the procedure is extremely safe and FDA-approved. All of the above treatments are lunchtime procedures and do not have significant downtime, but they should be carried out by qualified professionals only.

7. Can I do any skin treatments to prevent my hands from premature aging and at what age should I start?

Apart from basic hand care, one can get glycolic acid, lactic acid or mandelic acid peels once a month for about eight to ten sessions. This can be repeated every year. Microneedling with Dermapen is also a preventative anti-aging treatment. Hyaluronic acid skin booster injections are one of the best preventative anti-aging treatments for the hands. Hands are abused throughout the day. Hyaluronic acid booster injections help to maintain and retain moisture in the skin. They also repair the skin and rebuild the collagen, thus preventing fine lines and wrinkles. These treatments can be started at the age of thirty by all genders.

8. The skin around my fingertips and palms is always peeling. Sometimes it is very painful too. What can I do about this?

Do not peel the skin around your fingertips even if it seems to peel on its own. Use a gentle, soap-free body wash for bathing as well as washing your hands. Avoid the use of chalk and avoid gardening. Avoid hand sanitizers, Dettol or even regular handwashes as these can alter the skin pH and make it dry. This will lead to more skin peeling. Make sure you wear gloves whenever you wash clothes or utensils. Use a hand cream or thick, creamy moisturizer on your fingertips three to four times a day, especially after every wash. You may need a cream containing a corticosteroid if the peeling is severe or if you have developed eczema on your hands as a result of an allergy to soaps and detergents.

9. I have tiny bumps on my arms that are itchy at times, and they look horrible. What can I do to get rid of them?

You seem to be suffering from a condition called keratosis pilaris. These are seen as dark-coloured, raised bumps on the arms and sometimes on the legs and butt as well. The bumps are nothing but plugs of keratin, which is a protein. Sometimes they may be itchy, especially if the skin is dry. It is common in youngsters and is also common in those with atopic dermatitis, i.e., extremely dry skin. There is no cause identified and research has shown that it has an autosomal dominant mode of inheritance. You must use mild body washes and moisturize your skin two to three times a day. A 6 per cent salicylic acid lotion, 20 per cent urea cream,

10 per cent lactic acid or retinoids are usually prescribed to reduce keratosis pilaris. Lasers and microneedling have also been tried with limited improvement. There is no sure-shot treatment for keratosis pilaris.

10. I have extremely rough palms, though the rest of my hands and arms are smooth. I regularly moisturize my hands, but in vain. Could it be because of washing dishes? Please help.

Usually, repeated and prolonged exposure to soaps, detergents and handwashes damage the barrier layer of the skin, making it susceptible to allergies and infections and drying it out. You must try and avoid detergents. Use pH-balanced handwashes instead of soaps. Always moisturize your hands, especially after washing your hands. You may apply cooking oil or ghee before cutting vegetables or fruits as some of these are acidic and could irritate the skin further. Oil will form a good protective barrier on your skin. At bedtime, you must apply a generous coat of a thick moisturizer that has ceramides, which form the building blocks of our skin. Cocoa butter, shea butter, squalene and petrolatum are other ingredients you can look out for in your night cream.

FOOT CARE

Feet are small but they are the strongest. They bear the weight of our body and are true workhorses. Show them some TLC.

1. What are the basic steps for foot care?

Wash your feet with normal or lukewarm water and use a mild soap or body wash. Do not forget to clean the web spaces between your toes. After washing, dab the skin gently and apply a thick moisturizer. If you are going to wear slippers or sandals without socks, or if you remain barefoot, do not forget to apply a sunscreen over the moisturizer. At bedtime, apply a thicker moisturizer and wear cotton socks. Once or twice a week, you may use a pumice stone or a loofah and gently scrub the dead skin on the soles of your feet, especially the heels.

2. Is a pedicure a must for everyone?

A pedicure is a method for cleaning your toenails and the skin on the soles and feet. When you go to a salon it's more about pampering your skin, but you can also do a pedicure at home once a week. First trim your nails; do not dig into the corners and do not touch the cuticles. Then soak your feet in warm water for about five minutes. You must add a few drops of oil to the water. This will add moisture to the skin. Scrub all the dead skin away using a pumice stone, loofah or a brush, but be extremely gentle. Over-exfoliation can damage the protective layer of the skin. Use a gentle soap or shower gel to clean the feet. Rinse and dab gently. Apply a moisturizer containing shea butter or cocoa butter on slightly damp skin to lock the moisture within.

3. Why does one develop corns or calluses?

Calluses and corns are seen as thickened and hardened layers of skin on the soles of the feet. While calluses are just sheets of thick dead skin, corns are seen as inverted cones of hardened skin and are supplied by a blood vessel. Both occur on pressure-bearing areas of the foot and are more common on the pressure points that bear the maximum weight of the body. People with flat feet have higher chances of developing corns and calluses. Causes are friction, tight shoes, ill-fitting shoes, standing for long hours and frequent pedicures.

4. How does one treat and prevent corns and calluses?

Avoid tight and ill-fitting shoes and wearing high-heeled shoes for long hours. Preferably, opt for footwear that has a thick, cushioned sole. Wear a pair of socks or place gel pad inserts inside your shoes to avoid repeated friction and constant pressure on your soles. Existing calluses can be pared after cleaning the feet with soap water, and in the case of corns, salicylic acid ointment or lotion can be applied. If corns persist, one must consult a dermatologist or chiropodist as large corns require surgical excision.

5. I suffer from smelly feet. What is the remedy?

Smelly feet can occur due to excessive sweating, unclean, closed shoes, dirty socks or a fungal infection of the feet or soles. Excessive sweating can be genetic or can occur due to hormonal imbalance, or even certain medicines. While you can apply aluminium hydroxide hexahydrate solution, it works only temporarily. The other treatment is botulinum toxin injections into the soles of the feet. It is safe and the effect lasts for about six months, but it can be an expensive procedure.

Make sure you keep your feet clean and dry at all times. After washing your feet and drying them thoroughly, apply dusting powder or an antifungal powder such as Candid or Abzorb, especially on the soles and in the web spaces between the toes. Wear clean cotton socks and make sure you change your socks every day. Wash the socks in fragrance-free detergents and make sure the soap is thoroughly rinsed from the socks.

Avoid wearing closed shoes, and if you have to wear closed shoes to work, try and sun-dry them whenever possible. Avoid wearing the same pair of shoes on two consecutive days. Consult with a dermatologist to rule out fungal infections such as athlete's foot. Sweat combined with a dark environment, especially when one wears closed shoes, is a great breeding place for fungi and yeast. Prolonged use of tight-fitting shoes and socks can retain moisture in the web spaces of the feet, resulting in a candida infection. This is seen as a thick white layer between the toes. It may itch, especially at bedtime. Corynebacterial infections are seen on the soles, and athlete's foot can occur anywhere on the foot. Both are more common due to sweat or moisture retained due to prolonged wearing of socks and closed, tight shoes.

If you have a fungal infection or athlete's foot, your dermatologist will prescribe antifungal creams and oral medication usually for a course of two to three months. You must also follow the same principles of foot care every day.

6. What is athlete's foot? How can I prevent it as I am a runner?

Athlete's foot, also known as tinea pedis, is a fungal infection caused by a dermatophyte that also causes jock itch or ringworm. It does not occur only in athletes. It can occur in any individual and can cause itching, inflammation, cracks or a burning sensation on the feet. There could be various causes for athlete's foot. It could be due to persistent damp feet either due to sweating or prolonged wearing of closed shoes and damp socks. If one happens to share clothes, shoes, linen, towels, etc. with someone who has a fungal infection, one is likely to get athlete's foot. Walking barefoot in public areas such as dressing rooms of gymnasiums or playgrounds, swimming pool locker rooms, or communal bath and shower areas can also be another cause. Uncontrolled diabetes or high doses of steroid medication can also lead to athlete's foot.

To avoid athlete's foot, wash your feet twice a day and dry them properly. Take special care of the web spaces between the toes and always keep them dry. After bathing, use clotrimazole powder on your feet and dust some inside your shoes too. Make sure to wear clean and dry shoes and socks. Also, see to it that your shoes are breathable and the socks are mostly cotton that wick moisture. Avoid walking barefoot in public places.

If you already have athlete's foot, you may treat it by starting with the application of an antifungal cream containing clotrimazole or ketoconazole; however, make sure you consult a dermatologist immediately for proper medication. Do not neglect or self-treat the condition, especially with over-the-counter antifungal creams, which also contain steroids. This can lead to a resistant fungal infection, which becomes recurrent and extremely tough to treat.

7. Why does one develop cracked heels?

Cracked heels can be quite a pain, especially in winters. The various causes for cracked heels are washing the feet too often, especially with hot water, frequent use of lather-forming soap on the feet, wearing footwear such as slippers or sandals, dry, cold weather, prolonged standing, allergy to detergents, diabetes, hypothyroidism, obesity, fungal infection on the feet, flat feet, heel spurs, or bone protrusions on the bottom of your heel.

8. I have deep cuts and cracks on the soles of my feet, which increase in winter. No moisturizers help me. What should I do?

First of all, stop using regular soaps and shower gels. You must use a soap-free shower gel or syndet bar to wash your feet. Lather-forming soap can dry and damage the skin, aggravating the existing cracks on your soles.

Do not wash your feet obsessively. Too much water will dehydrate the skin. Wear cotton socks all the time, even during the day. Make sure you change your socks every day, and if possible, wear a different pair at night. Wash your socks using a fragrance-free detergent and ensure that all the soap is rinsed out. Any trace of soap in the socks that you wear can later mix with sweat and cause irritant contact dermatitis or allergic contact dermatitis. This may result in itching, burning, peeling and cracking of the skin. You must moisturize your feet two or three times in a day. Use moisturizers that contain occlusives, which seal the moisture into the skin and prevent trans-epidermal water loss from the skin. Also, use moisturizers with humectants, which draw water into the skin from the environment and from within the dermis. Emollients hydrate the skin and are equally important. Moisturizers containing ceramides also help repair the skin and prevent loss of moisture from the skin. At bedtime, use a moisturizer containing urea or lactic acid, which help remove dead skin. Opt for ointments or creams over lotions. In severe cases, consult a dermatologist.

9. What are the ingredients to look for in moisturizers?

It is best to have occlusives such as petrolatum, wax, oils and dimethicone; humectants such as hyaluronic acid, glycerin, urea, lactic acid, panthenol, honey and sorbitol; and emollients such as ceramides, fatty acids, cholesterol, shea butter and cocoa butter in your moisturizers.

10. My feet look very dark, especially my toes. The part where my footwear strap lies looks white as compared to

the rest of my feet. What can I do for this permanent tan that I have developed?

Your problem clearly seems to be sun-induced. Please apply a sunscreen on your feet every morning as a ritual even when you are indoors. At bedtime, you may use a cream containing skin lightening agents such as liquorice, kojic acid, arbutin, soy, glycolic acid, lactic acid, retinol, niacinamide and vitamin C. Do not forget to moisturize your skin twice a day. Chemical peels and pigment Lasers can be done at skin clinics to reduce hyperpigmentation that persists in spite of using creams and home remedies. Dark knuckles could occur due to obesity, acanthosis nigricans, pre-diabetes, diabetes, vitamin B12 deficiency, polycystic ovary syndrome (PCOS), scleroderma, Addison's disease and drug reactions. These conditions should be ruled out and treated as well.

11. I am developing corns on the soles of my feet. Corn caps are not helping. What should I do?

A corn is an patch of thickened skin that occurs in areas that are subjected to a lot of pressure. It is actually a normal and natural way for the body to protect itself. The problem occurs when the pressure continues, so the skin becomes thicker. It eventually becomes painful and is treated as something foreign by the body. Corns most commonly occur due to tight and improper footwear. Stop using corn caps. You can get the thickened surface of the corn pared and apply salicylic acid once or twice a week. If this doesn't help, you will have to get the corns removed surgically. Make sure you change your footwear and wear something soft and cushioned to prevent recurrence.

12. My job requires me to be on my feet for most of the day. As a result, I have calluses on my feet. They are very painful. Please help.

Wear shoes which give your toes plenty of room. If you are unable to wiggle your toes, your shoes are too tight for you and will cause pressure on your soles leading to callosities. Place a protective covering such as felt pads or gauze or a small bandaid over the callosity to decrease friction and/or pressure on the skin. Apply moisturizing agents with 10 per cent urea to soften the callosities and to make them easier to remove. Soak your feet in warm, soapy water and scrub the calluses with a pumice stone. You could also shave the hardened parts with a sterile blade. If the calluses do not reduce, they will need to be surgically removed by a doctor. You must wear soft, cushioned shoes to prevent recurrence.

13. I suffer from strawberry legs. Please tell me a way to get rid of them as I feel very embarrassed to wear shorts and skirts.

Strawberry legs are seen as tiny black dots on the legs. They usually occur when the pores get clogged with dead skin, bacteria and oil. Keratosis pilaris, ingrowth after shaving and folliculitis are other reasons for strawberry legs. Use salicylic acid, glycolic acid or retinol-based creams to cause chemo exfoliation. One may also opt for Laser hair removal or salicylic acid chemical peels to reduce the spots.

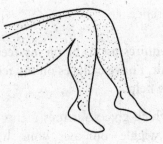

Applying a thick moisturizer helps reduce the appearance of strawberry legs if the skin is dry.

RAPID FIRE

1. I have black knuckles. Do I have to do a blood test to find out why?

Yes, please check your vitamin B12 levels.

2. My hands are peeling and they pain a lot. Will mustard oil help soothe my skin?

Mustard oil may further irritate the skin. Use coconut oil instead.

3. I have deep cuts and cracks on my feet. Is there a specific moisturizer I should use?

Apply a moisturizer with ceramides twice or thrice a day. This will repair the skin. In addition, you may also use a cream with urea twice a week, which will help to remove the dead skin gently.

4. My feet have gotten dark where the strap of my footwear touches my skin.

It can happen due to constant friction or due to allergy to the footwear material. Wear slightly loose footwear and change the material of the footwear.

5. When I wear socks, my feet stink. Otherwise they are fine.

Opt for cotton socks. Make sure you wash them with fragrance free detergents and dry them thoroughly. Dust some clotrimazole powder into your socks before wearing them.

12

Nail Care

'Beautiful nails are the best natural accessories of
your hands. Keep them neat.'

—Dr Jaishree Sharad

Nails are made of layers of keratin, a protein that is also
found in your hair and skin. The nail consists of a nail
plate, that is, the part that you trim and apply polish on.
Nail folds are the skin that borders your nail plate on
three sides. The nail bed is the skin just beneath the nail
plate. The cuticle is the protective layer between your
nail plate and the skin beneath your nails. Healthy nails
have pinkish-white nail plates and intact cuticles. Well-
groomed nails are a sign of beauty and they also add to
the youthfulness of the hands. Nails are a window to
some disorders of the internal organs of the body too.
Nails are an extension of the skin. Hence nail care should
be a part of your daily routine.

1. How do I take care of my nails?

Always keep your nails dry and clean. After washing your hands, make sure you rub a moisturizer not just on your hands but also on your nails. Never bite your nails. Trim your nails regularly using only a nail trimmer. While trimming them, be careful not to dig into the corners of the nails. Also, never cut the cuticles as they are meant to protect the nail bed from dirt, oil, bacteria and fungi. After trimming, file your nails with an emery board or a nail file and smoothen the corners. Do not leave any snags. Do not use acetone to remove nail polish. Avoid using your nails to open cans as that may damage your nails. If possible, while using soaps, detergents or any other harsh chemicals, wear waterproof rubber gloves.

2. Do toenails have to be treated differently than fingernails?

Both finger and toenail care remain the same. Always wear well-fitted shoes. When trimming your nails, smoothen the corners instead of digging into the skin. This will prevent the nail from growing into the skin. Nail fungus is more common in the toenails due to sweaty feet, dirty socks or wearing closed shoes for long hours. If you see your nails becoming yellow, consult with a dermatologist because this may be nail fungus, and it takes about six months of therapy for the nail to be completely free of fungus. Make sure you wear clean cotton socks and change your socks every day. Keep your feet dry at all times. If you wear closed shoes, try to remove them during your lunch hour and let your feet breathe.

3. How do you ensure your nails are healthy and strong?

Nails are made up of the protein keratin. It is important to have a diet rich in protein. Take supplements of amino acids, iron, magnesium, calcium, zinc, vitamin B especially vitamin B7, i.e., biotin, vitamins C and E, and omega 3 fatty acids. Avoid using toxic nail polishes and acetone to remove nail colour. Nail art, gel nails and acrylic nails indeed look beautiful and add glamour to your nails, but they make the nails brittle and deteriorate their quality and strength. Hence avoid getting them done very frequently. And give your nails a break at least once in two to three weeks. Avoid using glue on your nails frequently. Use nail hardeners sparingly and make sure you always moisturize your nails.

4. I'm suffering from ingrowing toenails. What is the remedy?

First of all, avoid wearing pointed or narrow shoes, which put a lot of pressure on your toenails. Instead, wear shoes with a wide toe box or wear open shoes. Do not cut the nails too short or dig into the corners to remove the nail that is growing into the skin. Consult a dermatologist in case of nail fungal infections or excessive sweating. Your dermatologist may even perform a toenail surgery known as partial nail avulsion with nail bed cauterization. However, remember to follow the steps of toenail care mentioned above to prevent recurrence even after surgery.

5. My nails look very yellow. Should I be concerned or is this normal?

Frequent use of nail polish can leave a yellowish hue on the nails. Fungal infections are the second-most common cause of yellow nails. It is advisable to consult a dermatologist to diagnose and treat the condition. Antifungal tablets, antifungal nail lacquers and lotions need to be used as per your dermatologist's prescription for six months in case of fingernail fungus and for up to twelve months in case of fungal infections of the toenails. Remember to keep your nails dry at all times.

6. My nails are very brittle and they keep breaking. Please help.

First, identify the cause of brittle nails and avoid the causes or treat them. Moisturize your nails at least two or three times a day. Take supplements of iron, calcium, magnesium, vitamin D3 and proteins.

7. Can I use acetone to remove my nail polish?

While acetone is a solvent and is the quickest way to remove nail polish, it is not the healthiest for our nails. Acetone can dehydrate the nail plate, cuticles and the surrounding skin. This can result in flaky, red, dry cuticles, inflammation of the surrounding skin and brittle nails over time. Opt for non-acetone polish removers instead. They contain ethyl acetate or n-methyl ethyl ketone and are gentler on the skin. It may take longer to remove the polish but it is safer. Some nail polish removers are also enriched with vitamin E, wheat germ oil, glycerine, etc. to add extra moisture to the nails and protect them. They are available as lotions or ready-to-use wipes, and are safe to use. Whether you use acetone- or non-acetone-based nail polish removers, always remember to moisturize your nails after removing nail polish.

8. Can I cut my cuticles since they look very worn out and ugly?

Cuticles protect the nail bed by sealing the gap between your skin and nails. This prevents the intrusion of dirt, bacteria and viruses into the nail bed and skin surrounding the nails. Cutting the cuticles may lead to bacterial, fungal and yeast infections of the nail and the skin around it. Paronychia, seen as a swollen, red, inflamed, painful nail with a lot of pus, is often a result of cutting the cuticles. So, one should always refrain from cutting the cuticles both at home and in a salon.

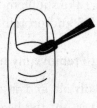

Avoid digging into cuticles

9. How safe is it to have artificial nails?

Artificial nails are of two types: acrylic and gel nails. Acrylic nails are long and can create a style statement. However, there is a downside to them. To apply the acrylic nail, one has to first file the surface of the natural nail and then use a glue to fix the acrylic nail to the natural nail. This makes the natural nail thin and weak. Some people may also be allergic to the glue. As your natural nails grow, gaps develop between the artificial nails and natural nails, which need to be filled every two to three weeks. These gaps can become breeding grounds for fungal or bacterial infections. Frequent touch-ups can seriously damage your natural nails, leaving them thin and brittle. Acrylic nails are removed by soaking the nails in acetone, which can again cause peeling and cracking of the natural nail.

Gel nails are another type of artificial nails in vogue. They are safer than acrylic nails. However, it is advisable to do minimal, mild buffing of the natural nail before applying the gel nail polish. Instead of using UV light to harden the gel nail, opt for LED lights, which emit a lower level of UV radiation and are safer for the skin. It is also advisable to apply a sunscreen on the entire length of the fingers and hands before exposing the nail to the LED lights.

10. Is it important to apply a base coat before applying nail polish?

A base coat forms a protective layer on the nail and prevents the nail from getting stained due to long nail polish wear. It also gives the nail a more even texture. Apply a base coat, allow it to completely dry and then apply a nail polish over it for best results. A base coat is a mixture of chemicals including solvents, resin, plasticizers etc. Some base coats also have vitamin A, vitamin E and calcium to help maintain the strength of the nail.

TYPES OF NAILS

- **Brittle nails:** Sometimes nails may break or chip very easily. Lack of nutrients such as proteins, calcium and vitamin D3, anaemia, low thyroid levels or hypothyroidism, Reynolds syndrome, frequent use of water, soaps and detergents, anti-cancer therapy or frequent use of acrylic or artificial nails can result in brittle nails.

- **Gnawed nails:** Nail-biting is known as onychotillomania in medical terms. This could just be a habit or a sign of persistent anxiety. Either way, it results in nail infections, paronychia and, of course, the nails don't look aesthetically pleasing. Sometimes you may develop gut infections as the nails may carry bacteria or fungi, which you can end up ingesting while biting your nails. Try to trim your nails short enough so you don't have room to bite them. Get a manicure regularly and, if you still can't stop the habit, it is better to seek help from a doctor.

- **Black toenails:** If you have a black toenail, you may have injured the nail; sometimes you may be unaware of the injury. Black nail is called a subungual hematoma in medical terms. Wearing tight shoes that cram your feet into the front of the shoe, stubbing a toe or someone stamping on your foot can injure a toenail resulting in a bruise. The bruise usually starts out red, then becomes bluish and finally black when the blood beneath the nail pools and clots. It usually takes six to twelve months for this to heal on its own.

- **Plummer's nail:** When a fingernail or a toenail separates from the nail bed either from the sides or the tip, it is called Plummer's nail or onycholysis. It usually occurs in the ring or little finger and is common in cases of hyperthyroidism. Dirt can easily collect beneath these nails and so can bacteria or yeast. Hence it is important to consult a dermatologist before the nail gets infected.

- **Spoon nails:** Nails that are concave and look like they have been scooped are seen in people suffering from hypothyroidism. So, if you see your nails looking like a spoon, it's time to get your thyroid hormones tested.
- **Blue nails:** Nails may appear blue in colour due to low oxygen, Raynaud's phenomenon, severe COVID-19 infection, a lung issue such as emphysema or heart failure.

RAPID FIRE

1. Are there any home remedies for nail care?

You can apply coconut oil or almond oil or even ghee to your nails and wear gloves overnight to hydrate the nails as well as the cuticles. Avoid using lime, vinegar and other acids on the nails.

2. I have white spots on my nails. Should I be worried?

You may sometimes see white spots on the nail plate, which may be a result of mild trauma to the nail bed. These are harmless and eventually grow out as the nail grows.

3. I have dark lines beneath the nail. What could it be?

Sometimes one may develop dark lines beneath the nails due to an injury to the nail or they could also be hints of melanoma, one of the most severe types of skin cancer. Consult a dermatologist.

4. My nail folds are very puffy. Why?

The folds of the nails may appear puffy due to a bacterial infection, lupus or connective tissue disorder.

5. My nails look yellow. What's the cause?

Nails may turn yellow in colour due to a fungal infection or prolonged wear of nail polish. Avoid wearing nail polish for a few days. If the yellowness persists, consult a dermatologist.

6. My nails look pale all the time. What's the reason?

Nails look pale due to anaemia, malnutrition, liver disease or congestive cardiac failure.

7. I have developed ripples on my nails. What should I do?

Nails may develop ripples on the surface due to psoriasis or inflammatory arthritis. Please consult a dermatologist.

8. Best Vitamin for nail?

Vitamin D3.

9. My friend doesn't use a nail cutter. He just bites his nails.

He may end up with bacterial or fungal infections.

10. Do I need to wash my nail clipper/cutter just like I wash my make up brushes ?

Most certainly yes!

13

Hair Care

'A woman who cuts her hair is about to change her life.'

—Coco Chanel

Hair is the crown one never takes off. Healthy, luscious hair is not just a sign of beauty but it also oozes confidence in all genders. My three-year-old niece was traumatized when her hair was shaved off as part of a religious ritual as much as her seventy-year-old grandfather who was traumatized due to balding as a natural process of aging. Good hair sees no age and it is important to start taking care of your hair from childhood.

On an average, each person's head carries about 1,00,000 hair follicles. Some people have as many as 1,50,000. Losing up to 100 strands of hair per day is normal. Each strand falls out eventually, and is replaced by a new one. Hair grows faster in summer and during sleep. Hair becomes drier with age. Hair is composed of keratin, which is resistant to wear and tear, fats, pigment (melanin), vitamins, zinc and other metals and water, which constitutes about 10 to 13 per cent of the hair. Hair care comprises health of hair, maintaining hygiene and hair cosmetics.

1. What are the steps of hair care?

Wash your hair two to four times a week depending on your scalp and hair type. Condition your hair to make it manageable. Use a wide-toothed comb or detangler to brush your hair after washing and drying it. Eat a high-protein, healthy diet.

2. Can we wash hair daily?

Yes, hair can be washed daily if you live in a polluted environment or sweat a lot. But use a mild shampoo if you have to wash your hair every day. Shampooing hair removes excess sweat, grime and any hair-styling products used. But shampooing too much can also strip the natural oils from the hair, making it dry and frizzy. If you have an oily scalp, you can wash your hair daily or on alternate days, but if you have extremely dry hair, then you must limit washing your hair to twice or thrice a week followed by conditioning.

3. Can oil be used for hair, and which is the best oil?

Coconut oil contains lauric acid, which has a high affinity for hair proteins and a low molecular weight, allowing the oil to penetrate to the cortex. Thus it is said to protect the hair shaft and prevent hair breakage or frizzy hair. Castor oil is rich in ricinolein, a monounsaturated fatty acid that allows it to act as a moisturizer. Argan oil has a high tocopherol and antioxidant capacity; however, there is a lack of scientific data on its efficacy with regard to hair conditioning. Almond oil contains high amounts of vitamin E, and is said to condition the hair shaft but lacks any scientific evidence.

Do not leave oil overnight in your hair. Wash your hair two to four hours after applying oil. Oil is a good conditioner and helps nourish the hair and reduce frizz. Regular oils that do not contain any added hair stimulating ingredients do not promote hair growth or stop hair fall.

4. What should one eat for healthy hair?

Hair is made of keratin, which is primarily a protein, acids and amino acids. For healthy lustrous hair, one should have a diet rich in protein, iron, zinc, selenium, calcium, amino acids, collagen, magnesium, folic acid, omega 3 fatty acids, vitamins A, D, E, C, B3 and B12, and biotin.

5. Should we use a conditioner after washing the hair?

Application of hair conditioners after shampooing will lower inter-fibre friction and reduce combing force and static electricity. A conditioner nourishes the hair, makes it softer and more manageable, and increases shine.

M.F. Gavazzoni Dias. Hair Cosmetics: An Overview. *International Journal of Trichology*. 2015; 7 (1): 2–15. doi:10.4103/0974-7753.153450.

It is especially required for hair that has undergone chemical or heat treatments, or has turned dry, frizzy and unmanageable. Always apply a conditioner along the length of the hair shaft and never on the scalp. Make sure you rinse the conditioner well unless it is a leave-in conditioner.

6. Does plucking a grey hair cause several more grey hair strands to grow in its place?

Hair changes with age, the same way as our skin shows signs of aging. As we age, follicles produce less melanin due to which our hair starts to lose its colour and turns grey or white. Other reasons due to which hair shows early signs of aging are stress, an unhealthy diet, smoking, environmental factors, various hair treatments, hormonal imbalance or nutritional deficiency. On plucking grey hair, the new hair that grows will be white or grey because the melanin-producing cells in the hair root and its surrounding area have died. Which is why, sometimes, more hair that grow from this area of the scalp will be white or grey.

7. Do we need any special care for wet hair?

Do not wrap a towel too tight over the scalp. Avoid vigorous towel drying as traction can cause friction and hair loss. Do not use a fine-bristled comb. Wide-toothed hair detanglers are better as they will not cause hair breakage. Wet hair when tied is a harbour for fungi, bacteria, yeast and even lice. Never tie your hair when it is damp. Dry your hair before tying. Use an air dryer instead of hair dryer. Try using warm or cold air from a distance instead of using hot air with a temperature above 150 degrees.

8. How can one reduce hair damage?

Practise proper hair-care methods. Avoid keeping your hair tied for long periods of time, be it in a bun or tight ponytail, or parting the hair in the same direction and area over years. Avoid styling the hair with harsh products and the continuous use of hair products. Know your hair type and hair requirements and use products accordingly. Have a healthy, protein-rich diet.

9. How does one treat lice?

You should apply permethrin lotion on the scalp for about ten minutes and then wash your hair. Do this thrice a week for about three weeks. Dry your hair completely before you tie it up. A lice infestations is easily passed from person to person in the same house, hence members of the family may need treatment for lice infestation to prevent lice from coming back. Lice are spread by the head or body-to-body contact, storing clothing such as scarves or storing personal items such as pillows, blankets, combs, brushes and stuffed toys of infected and non-infected persons in close proximity.

Wash clothing and bed linens in very hot water to kill the lice and their eggs. Hair-care items such as combs and brushes can either be soaked in hot water or medicated shampoo or thrown away. Brush your hair thrice a day to get rid of the dead nits and lice.

10. What are the causes of dandruff?

Dandruff could occur due to a change in climate, hormonal imbalance, a product applied to your hair or even stress. These trigger excessive secretion of sebum and a build-up of dead cells on the scalp. The scales along with sebaceous secretions tend to stick to the scalp and together make up the common condition known as dandruff. This may or may not be itchy. Studies have revealed that a type of fungus, called Malassezia, which lives naturally on the scalp of many people, increases at times and leads to dandruff. Infection, an injury to the scalp, faulty diet and excessive use of hair cosmetics such as sprays, gels, etc. can also cause dandruff.

11. Please suggest a permanent remedy for dandruff. No amount of curd or lime juice seems to help and it gets worse during winters.

There may be no permanent solution for dandruff if it is the result of an inflammatory disorder of the scalp. You should keep your hair and scalp clean and dry. Use a shampoo with zinc pyrithione and ketoconazole. Tea tree oil-based shampoos are also good options for mild dandruff. Avoid heat treatments or frequent blow-drying. If the dandruff is persistent, you can use a shampoo that has coal tar in it once a week. If you have a flaky scalp, you must not use a heavy conditioner, hair oil or hair serum. Avoid applying oil since you already have an oily scalp. If the dandruff does not subside with the above care, please consult a dermatologist as you may be suffering from seborrheic dermatitis or psoriasis of the scalp, both of which are inflammatory scalp disorders.

12. Can you suggest a home remedy for dandruff?

Rub a mixture of curd and crushed fenugreek seeds on the scalp, keep it on for ten minutes and then rinse. Do this twice a week. Mild-to-moderate dandruff does reduce with this simple home remedy.

13. I have dry, scaly patches on my scalp, eyebrows and eyelids. They are very itchy. What should I do?

You are probably suffering from seborrhoeic dermatitis. It usually aggravates in winter and if you are under stress. Please consult a dermatologist. Use a 2 per cent ketoconazole-based shampoo twice a week. Do not stay in an air-conditioned room for long hours and do not take hot showers. For your brows, you may apply petroleum jelly.

14. Winters make our skin dry and rough. How can one protect the eyelids? Also, I develop a white patch and collarettes on the top lid. What can be done for this?

Flaky eyelids are common in winter due to a condition known as seborrhoeic dermatitis. Apply ketoconazole cream on the eyelid skin once a day. Apply a drop of coconut oil twice a day and avoid harsh soaps and face washes. This will help reduce the dryness on the lids.

15. Can eggs be used as conditioners? How can one use them?

Yes, eggs can be used as conditioners. Just be prepared for the smell that persists on the scalp post the use of eggs. Eggs are full of proteins, and they revitalize the hair while cleaning it. Shampoo your scalp. Then, beat one or two eggs, add a cup of water and massage this into your wet hair continuously for about ten minutes. Rinse off thoroughly. Don't use hot water. As a last rinse, you can use the juice of one lemon in a cup of lukewarm water.

16. I have always had straight hair but now it is becoming curly. What could be the reason? I have not permed my hair.

An increase in androgens (male hormones) in females due to a hormonal imbalance can actually change the shape of the hair follicle from round to flat and this can instigate a change in texture from straight to curly.

17. I have curly hair, and it has become too frizzy to manage. How can I tame my hair?

Use a mild shampoo and good conditioner that won't weigh the hair down yet condition it. You must avoid using heat-styling tools to prevent damage to the hair. Regular deep conditioning of the hair at a hair studio can give it a healthier bounce and shine. Use good detangling products and a wide-toothed comb for the hair. Avoid frequent blow-drying. Opt for an air-dryer if possible. If not, then try gentle towel drying. Use a nourishing hair cream or gel in small quantities to keep your hair non-frizzy and straight.

18. I recently coloured my hair but had an allergic reaction to the colour. My skin is now inflamed, swollen and burning. How do I treat this?

You must consult a dermatologist. You may need a medicated solution containing cortisone. In the meantime, take an anti-allergy tablet like fexofenadine. Avoid any hair colour or hair dye. You are most probably allergic to PPD, an essential ingredient in most chemical hair colours. Opt for vegetable dyes or PPD-free organic colours instead. Natural hair dyes prepared from Indian gooseberry (Emblica officinalis), false daisy (Eclipta alba), lotus tree (Ziziphus spina-christi) and henna (Lawsonia alba) are hypoallergenic and non-toxic and can be tried.

19. My hair is really brittle and gets split ends just weeks after a trim. What can I do to make it stronger?

Split ends occur when the cuticle is removed from the hair shaft, and the soft keratin cortex and medulla are exposed to weathering, leading to formation of cracks in the hair fibre and split ends. Sunlight, physical trauma to the hair shaft caused due to vigorous combing, excessive shampooing, drying or brushing, or chemical damage by bleaches, dyes or straighteners can lead to split ends. Avoid the cause. Use a conditioner or leave-in serum after every wash. Get the existing split ends trimmed. You must have a diet rich in proteins and take supplements of iron and zinc to strengthen your hair.

20. My daughter is ten years old and is suffering from heavy hair loss. What can I do?

Hair loss in a child is usually the result of a nutritional deficiency, unless she suffered from an illness six to ten weeks ago, which could result in the condition called telogen effluvium when one sheds hair. Give her a diet rich in proteins, iron and calcium. Get her haemoglobin and vitamins B12 and D3 levels checked. She should be given supplements if these are found to be deficient.

You can also consult with her paediatrician and give her supplements of vitamins A, B and C and some minerals. Use a mild shampoo and conditioner twice a week. If this doesn't help, you must get her hair and scalp examined by a dermatologist.

21. I am in my early thirties and have been getting a lot of grey hair. Please tell me how to stop this and how I can make the grey hair black again.

Premature greying of hair can be genetic and occur as an autosomal dominant primary disease. Oxidative stress (oxidative stress is a phenomenon caused by an imbalance between production and accumulation of oxygen-reactive species [ROS] in cells and tissues and the ability of a biological system to detoxify these reactive products) influences the hair follicle stem cells and damages the melanocytes (a cell in the skin which produces pigment melanin) in the hair root leading to decreased pigmentation and greying. Exposure to ultraviolet rays, pollution, emotional factors, a prolonged illness or autoimmune disorders such as hypothyroidism or vitiligo can increase oxidative stress, leading to premature hair greying. Deficiency of vitamins D3 and B12, copper, iron, calcium and zinc also leads to greying of hair. Smoking causes increased reactive oxygen species damage (damage to the basic building blocks of the cell including DNA, protein and lipids) to hair follicle melanocytes and results in greying.

While complete reversal may not be possible, identifying the cause and treating it is the first step towards treatment. Supplements of iron, calcium, zinc, copper and vitamins B12 and D3 will help. Quit smoking if you are a smoker. Learn to cope with stress. Serums containing green tea extract, selenium, copper, phytoestrogens and melatonin are being studied to reverse hair greying with minimum results as of today. A new type of compound (SkQs) comprising an antioxidant known as plastoquinone SkQs, has been shown to inhibit age-related changes such as canities, retinopathy, cataract, etc. Liposomal delivery of melanin into hair follicles through mesotherapy has resulted in darkening of hair follicles.

22. I am a twenty-year-old male. I am losing a lot of hair and have developed a bald patch on my crown. My dad became bald at the age of sixty, so it can't be genetic. What should I do?

You seem to be suffering from male pattern or androgenetic alopecia. It usually starts at the temples, leaving an M pattern on the forehead and then spreads to the crown and occiput. It's almost always genetic, and even though your dad started balding at the age of sixty, you have a genetic predisposition. Extrinsic factors such as stress, pollution and an unhealthy lifestyle can lead to early balding.

You should consult with a dermatologist or trichologist and get a trichoscopy done. Get your haemoglobin, calcium, vitamins B 12 and D3 and thyroid hormones tested. Hair is made up of keratin, which is nothing but protein and amino acids. Your daily protein intake should

A.B. Kumar, H. Shamim, U. Nagaraju. Premature Graying of Hair: Review with Updates. *International Journal of Trichology*. 2018; 10 (5): 198–203. doi:10.4103/ijt.ijt_47_18Urentebus, C. Ut L. Senatemo ubli pubiti corem imis vivera be at least 1 gram per kilo of body weight. The medicines approved by the US Food and Drug Administration for male pattern alopecia are minoxidil solution, finasteride and dutasteride. While minoxidil has to be used for life, those who are allergic to minoxidil can opt for topical solutions containing capixyl, peptides, azelaic acid or tretinoin, which will also promote hair growth. In the initial phases of male pattern or female pattern balding, mesotherapy and platelet-rich plasma treatment also promote hair regrowth.

23. What is a hair cycle?

The growth of the hair follicle is cyclical. Stages of rapid growth and elongation of the hair shaft alternate with periods of quiescence and regression.

Stages of male pattern balding

The hair cycle comprises:
Anagen – growth phase, which lasts for two to six years. It is the active phase in which the hair follicle takes on its onion-like shape and works to produce the hair fiber.

Catagen – involution phase, which usually lasts for two weeks. During this phase, the hair follicle undergoes regression and loses about one-sixth of its standard diameter.

Telogen – resting phase, which lasts for one to three months. Normally, 10 to 15 per cent of a person's hair is in the telogen phase at any one time. In this cycle, hair follicle is dormant, and growth of the hair shaft does not occur.

24. I am a forty-nine-year-old female and am balding in the front. My parting is getting wider though I do not see much hair fall.

You seem to be suffering from female pattern alopecia, which involves shortening of the anagen cycle of the hair. The hair follicle also shrinks in size and the hair shaft becomes shorter and thinner. This process is called 'follicular miniaturization'. According to the Ludwig Classification for female pattern hair loss, Type I is minimal thinning that can be camouflaged with hair styling techniques. Type II is characterized by decreased volume and noticeable widening of the central parting. Type III is characterized by diffuse thinning, with a see-through appearance on the top of the scalp. While the underlying cause is genetic, hormonal imbalances such as hypothyroidism, hyperthyroidism, PCOS and insulin resistance are known to increase female pattern alopecia. Treatment includes topical minoxidil, oral finasteride or dutasteride in older females as well as Aldactone and flutamide in younger females. Please do not take any of these medicines on your own. They need to be prescribed by a dermatologist. A healthy, stress-free lifestyle, high-protein diet and avoiding smoking are equally important.

25. I suffered from COVID-19 in the first week of January 2022. I have been experiencing a lot of hair fall since March. Is it related to COVID? Is there a treatment? Will my hair grow back? I am only twenty-seven years old.

Illnesses such as COVID-19, malaria, dengue, swine flu or tuberculosis, surgery, trauma, pregnancy, stress, poor diet, crash diets, starvation, sudden weight loss, certain drugs or the wrong hair treatments can release the anagen hair into the telogen phase at a rapid rate, leading to hair shedding. This condition is called telogen effluvium. It usually starts six to ten weeks after the triggering episode. It takes about four to six months for the telogen hair to shed completely and for the anagen hair to grow back. Clumps of hair with the entire bulb (whitish tip) are shed, leaving the person anxious.

You are suffering from acute telogen effluvium post COVID. Please consult a dermatologist, who will prescribe the right supplements and hair serums to treat your condition. The good thing is that telogen effluvium does not cause baldness. With proper medication, supplements and diet, almost all the hair grows back.

26. I was prescribed minoxidil for hair loss. I started losing more hair after using it. Does minoxidil cause impotence? And will my hair fall more after stopping minoxidil?

With minoxidil, the anagen phase of hair cycle is initiated. Thus, the exogen hair, which were resting, begin to shed two to eight weeks after starting minoxidil. This is normal, paradoxical hair fall and will stop as soon as all the exogen hair fall out. So, continue to use the minoxidil.

Minoxidil is approved by the US Food and Drug Administration and is a well-researched molecule with significant results. It does not cause impotence or any such side effects. It may cause headaches sometimes, especially if the formulation is alcohol-based. The anagen phase may go back to being short once you stop minoxidil, and your hair fall will begin again. But minoxidil is not the culprit. Just as you take medicines for a heart ailment for life, you have to use minoxidil for life if the hair fall is due to male pattern or female pattern alopecia.

27. I have done rebonding a couple of times, and my hair is now breaking a lot and has become brittle and dry. What can I do to stop this?

When damp hair is subjected to a lot of heat during treatments such as straightening, ironing, rebonding and perming, the water inside the hair shaft is heated and turns into steam. This results in bubble hair which is a hair shaft abnormality. Hair bubbles collect on the hair shaft and damage the hair cuticle and hair structure. This results in frizzy hair, dry, fly-away hair, hair breakage and thinning of hair.

Make sure you use shampoos and conditioners meant for straightened/permed/rebonded hair. Use a conditioner after every shampoo. Dimethicone reduces static electricity and improves manageability of hair. So, it's a good idea to look for dimethicone as an ingredient in your shampoos, conditioners and serums. Avoid hair dyes and go for hair colour instead. Always opt for a dark colour. A lighter shade will require bleaching of the natural hair, which can be harmful. Whenever possible, allow the hair to air dry. Avoid vigorous towel drying or using hot air blow-dryers every day. If you need to, use a cold air dryer instead of a hot one. Moisturize your hair by applying leave-in hair serums to the hair and not the scalp. If you have to use a ceramic iron to straighten your hair, use a heat-protecting spray on the hair shaft before ironing. If you have had keratin or cysteine treatments done, you could end up with similar hair breakage and frizzy hair issues if the aftercare is not proper.

Avoid frequent treatments and always wash your scalp well and then condition the ends of your hair. If the hair becomes too frizzy, wait till you get new hair growth. Wear a hat to protect hair from ultraviolet rays. And last but not the least, increase your protein intake to strengthen your hair. Take supplements of iron, biotin, amino acids and minerals to increase hair density and quality.

28. I have very oily hair and I also workout and sweat a lot in my scalp. I want to shampoo daily, but I'm afraid my hair will start falling. What should I do?

Sweat and sebum on the scalp will attract more dust, dirt and grime and make the scalp susceptible to infections. In order to maintain scalp hygiene, it is better to shampoo daily if you have a very oily scalp or sweat excessively on the scalp. Use a mild shampoo and conditioner. Avoid heat treatments to the hair.

29. I have been told that hair shouldn't be combed when it is wet. But my hair knots easily.

When the hair is wet, water penetrates the hair shaft, so it swells and starts tangling with other hair. If wet hair is not combed, it will dry out tangled, making it unmanageable and difficult to style. So, it is better to use a wide-toothed detangler and gently comb your hair when they are wet. Apply a serum to the hair shaft. This way you will prevent knots.

30. What are the reasons for hair loss?

There are plenty of causes of hair loss, namely:
- Genetic, which can lead to male pattern or female pattern alopecia
- Stress, which can release hormones that reduce the anagen phase and lead to hair shedding
- An infection such as COVID-19, malaria, dengue, tuberculosis, typhoid, etc.; surgery or trauma; diseases such renal failure or a liver disorder; or starvation or crash diets can all cause telogen effluvium
- Nutritional deficiency, especially proteins, vitamins A, B, C, D and E, biotin, iron, calcium, zinc, chromium and magnesium
- Hormonal imbalances such as those caused by hypothyroidism, hyperthyroidism, PCOS, a pituitary disorder, menopause, post-pregnancy, etc.
- Drug-induced, for example, patients on anti-cancer treatment, anti-thyroid drugs, cholesterol-lowering agents and patients on anticoagulant therapy suffer from hair loss

- Frequent heat treatments such as ironing, straightening, etc., if not done properly
- Scalp diseases or infections such as psoriasis or severe folliculitis
- Trichotillomania, a disorder in which the person pulls out his/her hair from the scalp, eyelashes or eyebrows intentionally
- Immense traction on the hair roots when the hair is tied into a tight ponytail or certain hair braiding styles can cause traction alopecia
- Autoimmune disorders such as alopecia areata

31. What are the dos and don'ts for patients with hair loss?

Use a mild shampoo depending on the hair type (normal, dry or oily) and do not forget to condition your hair. A diet rich in proteins, iron and zinc should be consumed. Include whole grains, pulses, sprouts, egg white, chicken, lean meat, milk, soya, tofu and mushrooms in your diet. Take supplements of vitamins A, B, C and E, biotin, zinc, calcium, magnesium, chromium, selenium and omega 3 fatty acids. Check your haemoglobin, vitamins D3 and B12 and replenish if deficient. Get all your hormone and other relevant blood tests done. Psychological stress and anxiety lead to hair loss, so learn to cope with stress. Physical trauma to the hair shaft caused due to vigorous combing, excessive shampooing, drying or brushing should be avoided. Beware of trendy styles, hair bleaching and dyeing as they might cause more harm than good. Avoid hair perming or straightening, hair botox, cysteine and keratin treatments.

32. What are the best shampoos for dandruff?

You can use any anti-dandruff shampoo that contains medicated ingredients such as selenium sulphide, which is an antifungal agent; imidazole antifungal agents such as ketoconazole, which kills the dandruff-causing fungi; hydroxypyridones such as ciclopirox and pyrithione zinc, which are antifungal; salicylic acid, which eliminates scales; and piroctone olamine, which is antimicrobial and antifungal and promotes hair growth. Washing three times a week enables the dead corneocytes to be removed, decreases oiliness of the scalp and helps clear dandruff. Always apply the anti-dandruff shampoo on a slightly wet scalp, leave it on for at least fifteen minutes to facilitate proper penetration of the ingredients and then rinse it.

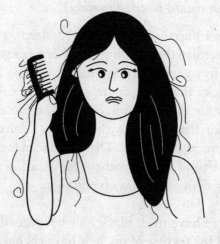

33. How can I reduce the frizz in my hair? Does oiling help?

Frizzy hair is the result of a dry scalp due to exposure to sun, heat or pollution, or a natural process of aging, or damaged cuticles due to frequent heat styling treatments.

First of all, avoid anything to do with heat and hair. Use a hyaluronic acid, dimethicone or glycerine rich conditioner to hydrate the hair shaft. These are humectants; they absorb extra moisture in the air, lock in the moisture and form a protective coating over the hair shaft. They also seal the cuticles. Use a hair mask once a week. Oiling once a week will also reduce frizz. You can also use a leave-in serum. Air drying wet hair and sleeping on silk pillow cases help too.

34. How are hair masks different from conditioners and serums with regard to conditioning?

Hair masks are applied on the scalp for deep conditioning. They are useful in those with severely dry, frizzy, damaged or chemically treated hair. Hair masks or packs are usually protein packs that may contain silicones, collagen and quaternary ammonium compounds. The protein diffuses into the hair shaft through the cuticular defects created by the chemical treatment. The protein adds strength to the hair shaft and also smoothens the cuticular scale more thoroughly than an instant conditioner.

35. I used to have thick black hair but recently both the colour and the texture of my hair have changed. My hair is now brown and straw-like in appearance. My work is usually outdoors. Could that be the reason?

Hair gets bleached on exposure to UV rays as well as visible light. The protein cysteine in the hair cuticle gets damaged too. This leads to a change in the colour and texture of the hair. Use a good hair serum to form a protective coat on your hair cuticle. Wear a UV-protective a dark-coloured scarf or bandana to cover your hair when outdoors. Grey and white hair are more susceptible to UV damage than black or brown hair. Also, the rate of cystine disulfide bond breakage is greater for unpigmented than pigmented hair. So, a dark-coloured hair dye or hair colour can also form a protective coat over your hair.

36. Can hair colour cause hair fall?

Good-quality hair colour will not cause hair fall. Extremely frequent use of hair colour may cause the hair to become dry or brittle. Always use shampoos and conditioners meant for colour-treated hair. Avoid bleaching your hair as far as possible. Opt for darker hair colours if possible. Ammonia-free colours and vegetable dyes are safer.

37. What are hair serums? How does one use a serum?

Hair serums are styling products that can be used to treat dull or frizzy hair, and to prevent heat damage. Silicone-based serums protect the hair shaft and reduce frizz.

Add one to two drops of hair serum to the palm of your hand and apply to clean, damp hair.

Work from the ends up to the middle of the hair strands. Avoid applying the serum to your hair roots. Avoid using too much product, as this can make your hair look greasy.

Use a wide-tooth comb to gently distribute the serum evenly from the middle of your strands down to the ends.

38. Does onion juice help in hair growth?

Onion juice can irritate the scalp and may cause a reaction, irritant contact dermatitis or scarring. It is better to avoid such remedies and consult a dermatologist instead. Onion juice causes inflammation in an autoimmune condition called alopecia areata where one develops circular, well defined patches of hair loss. The irritation to the scalp in alopecia areata may sometimes stimulate the hair roots and result in some hair regrowth. But there is no scientific evidence to support this, and it is better to seek proper treatment from a doctor.

39. Does platelet-rich plasma therapy help in hair regrowth or is stem cell therapy a better option?

Platelet-rich plasma or PRP therapy involves collection of one's own blood, centrifugation and collection of platelet-rich plasma. This PRP is rich in growth factors, cytokines and platelets, which will stimulate the stem cells and hair follicles to regenerate. It is injected into the bald patches on the scalp. Usually six to eight sessions are done at monthly intervals for hair regrowth. It is a safe lunchtime procedure and can be done by anyone less than fifty years with hair thinning or hair loss. One gets better results with stem cells but stem cell therapy is a more invasive and tedious procedure. In the stem cell procedure, a mini-liposuction is performed on the abdomen to obtain one to two ounces of adipose (fat) tissue. Using special on-site equipment, stem cells are then extracted from the fat sample, combined with the PRP, and injected into the scalp.

40. When should one opt for a hair transplant?

When a person has severe androgenetic alopecia, significant hair thinning or cicatricial alopecia and is not responding to medical treatment, a hair transplant is the only option. Patients with Norwood grade VI or VII with poor hair density are not good candidates for a hair transplant.

41. I have very thin eyelashes. I don't like wearing false eyelashes as they look fake. Is there a way that I can naturally get thicker eyelashes?

Bimotropsot serum helps increase both the length and thickness of lashes. Also, there are certain serums that help in the growth of lashes. Your dermatologist may prescribe them for you. You will have to use the medication for three to four months for a satisfactory result. Avoid using mascara if you have thin eyelashes. Take enough proteins in your diet and biotin supplements as well. If you had thick lashes and they become scanty suddenly, you must consult a dermatologist as there is a possibility that you may be suffering from alopecia areata.

42. I am considering going in for microblading of eyebrows. Are there any side effects?

First of all, get the procedure done by a professional who is well trained and also has an artistic eye. The shape of the eyebrows should match the face. Second, the instrument, ink and blade should be sterile and the procedure should be performed under hygienic sterile conditions. Good-quality ink should be used. Unlike tattoo ink, which is made of iron oxide and is dispersible, microblading inks are non-dispersible. Good quality microblading inks are non-magnetic, organic and do not contain any heavy metals. Microblading inks usually develop a blackish-greyish tinge with repeated sun exposure. Hence touch-ups are needed.

Asymmetry, unnatural shape or change of colour are the cosmetic side effects of microblading. Sometimes, there is temporary pain and bruising. More serious side effects such as infections, especially mycobacterial and herpes, or granuloma formations can occur if the equipment is not sterile or poor quality ink is used. Spread of HIV and HBS Ag occurs if blades are shared.

43. I am a flight attendant and take good care of my skin and hair. In spite of that, my hair feels very dry and frizzy, especially in the winter. What extra care can I take to make it more manageable?

Dryness of the skin and hair is common in winter. This along with long hours in an air-conditioned atmosphere will further exacerbate dryness and make your hair frizzy. Use warm water while shampooing your hair. Warm water opens the hair cuticles and helps to absorb conditioner, which goes directly to your hair shaft (root) and treats it by moisturizing. Do not forget to use cool water while rinsing out the conditioner. This will close your hair cuticles again and will help prevent more frizz. Use a good moisturizing conditioner containing vitamin E, aloe vera, peptides, proteins and panthenol after shampooing your hair. Leave it in for three to five minutes. Avoid too much brushing and blow-drying as this will rip the moisture from your hair and cause more frizz. Avoid hair treatments such as ironing, perming and straightening as far as possible. If done, you must see that you use a leave-in conditioner or an anti-frizz hair serum after every wash. Have sunflower seeds, flax seeds, pumpkin seeds, walnuts, almonds, avocado and supplements of omega 3 fatty acids.

44. Are sulphate shampoos bad for the hair?

Sulphates are cleansing agents present in shampoos. They cleanse the hair of grease, grime, sebum, sweat salts, dead skin, dirt, oil, hair products and debris. If your scalp and hair are normal, greasy or oily, it is fine to use sulphate-based shampoos. If you have a sensitive scalp or have had multiple heat treatments leading to dull and brittle hair, sulphates may strip the extra oil making the scalp and hair drier. So, it is best to know your hair type and use a shampoo suited for it.

RAPID FIRE

1. My twelve-year-old son has severe hairfall. What's the reason?

Any illness, truma, acute stress or a nutritional deficiency may lead to hair fall.

2. I can see small bald patches on my fifteen-year-old daughter's scalp. The doctor said it is not alopecia areata which I had read up online.

Sometimes children pull their hair as a habit or due to anxiety. The condition is called trichotillomania. Please get it checked by a dermatologist.

3. Which is the one wonder vitamin for hair?

Unfortunately, there in no 'single' wonder vitamin for hair. You need vitamins, mineral, trace elements and proteins for good hair.

4. Will I have more hair fall if I shampoo my hair daily?

Not at all. Just use a mild shampoo or baby shampoo.

5. Will I get more hair if I brush my hair hundred times a day?

This is a myth. In fact, brushing your hair so many times may make your hair brittle and damage your hair shaft

6. Will my hair grow long if I trim it from time to time?

Trimming will get rid of split ends but will have no effect on the length of your hair.

7. My hair gets used to a shampoo. How should I choose my shampoo?

Hair never get used to a shampoo. Either your scalp has gotten oilier or dry due to hormones or hair products you have used or due to chemical treatments like coloring, rebonding etc. Hence the shampoo needs to be changed.

8. How often do I need to apply oil to hair?

You can oil your hair once a week and leave it in for about two hours before shampooing.

9. Should serums be used?

Yes, a hair serum can be used, especially if you have dry hair. Also, applying a serum before using hair-styling products protects the hair.

10. What is a safe way to blow-dry hair?

Use the lowest setting on your blow dryer and hold it at least 6 inches away from your hair. Do not hold the dryer on any one spot for too long as that can heat the hair and damage the shaft. Instead, keep moving your dryer continuously.

14

Face and Body Hair Removal

'Unwanted body hair is unnecessary extra
maintenance, get rid of it.'

—Dr Jaishree Sharad

Cleopatra, the Queen of Egypt, is said to have believed that
having body hair was an indicator of being 'uncivilized'.
Around 3000 BC, Ancient Egyptians used tweezers,
sugar scrubs, a mixture of burnt lotus leaf, tortoiseshell
and hippo fat, and pumice stones to remove all hair from
their body, except for their eyebrows.

In the Roman era (around 400 BC), it was said that
the amount of hair on a woman's body was inversely
proportional to one's status in society.

Around the 1500s, in England, mothers from wealthy
families would rub walnut oil, and the less economically
privileged would put bandages soaked in ammonia (which

they obtained from their feline pets' faeces) on their daughters' foreheads to prevent hair growth.

Body hair removal is now a very common protocol both for hygiene and cosmetic purposes in all genders. Various methods from shaving to Lasers are used for hair removal.

1. Is it safe to use ubtan or a pumice stone on babies to remove hair from their bodies?

Body hair in infants is known as lanugo hair, and it falls out on its own; one doesn't need to do anything special to remove it. Ubtan can lead to folliculitis or infantile acne. Pumice stone can irritate the skin and can even cause post-inflammatory hyperpigmentation. It is better to allow the hair to fall out on its own. If the condition persists even after the child is five years old, it is better to consult a paediatric endocrinologist to rule out an endocrine condition.

2. I am a twenty-three-year-old female. Is it okay to shave my facial hair ?

It is absolutely okay to shave your facial hair. Follow these steps and you won't have any problem shaving. Make sure you use a new blade; it should be sharp. Dip your razor or trimmer in hot water before shaving and wash your face well. Remove all make-up from your face. Use a good-quality shaving cream or foaming soap and forms a good lather on the face. Do not do a dry shave as you can end up with razor bumps. Once you form a lather, stretch your skin and then shave in the direction of the hair growth, i.e., along the direction of the grain. This will prevent ingrown hair and acne. After you shave, wash your face with warm water and apply an antibacterial cream, aloe vera gel or any soothing gel that will calm your skin.

3. What are the side effects of shaving?

The hair grows back very quickly and the skin feels rough when there is a stubble. If you shave in the direction opposite to the hair growth, i.e., against the grain, then you have a greater chance of developing ingrown hair or razor bumps. You may develop folliculitis if the razor blade is dirty or infected with bacteria.

4. What is the difference between folliculitis and razor bumps?

Folliculitis is an infection of the hair follicle caused by bacteria, especially staphylococcus aureus. They are seen as tiny, yellow-coloured, pus-filled boils. Razor bumps are ingrown hair seen as bumps on the skin, sometimes with a black tip.

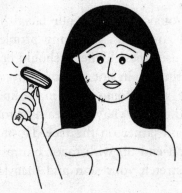

5. I always develop ingrown hair after shaving or waxing. What should I do?

When hair is pulled, sometimes part of the hair curls and grows into the skin, leading to bumps or ingrown hair. Sometimes these get infected and lead to folliculitis. Other times they are seen as tiny black bumps on the skin surface.

Ingrown hair or pseudo folliculitis barbae or razor bumps can be prevented by following the correct method of shaving. Antibacterial creams and retinol or AHA/BHA-based creams are prescribed to reduce ingrown hair. Aloe vera gel and warm compresses are used to soothe the skin. Sometimes one may have to extract the hair from beneath the skin. A permanent and best solution, however, is Laser hair removal.

6. Is epilation a good method of hair removal? Can I epilate my hair regularly?

Epilation is a simple and effective form of temporary hair removal that can be done by all genders and age groups. An epilator is a small, handheld device that has multiple sets of tweezers on a roller. As the roller rotates, the tweezers grab your hairs and remove them from the root. You can remove very short hairs with epilators. The hair does not grow back fast because it is pulled out from the roots. Epilators come with attachments for various parts of the body such as the face, eyebrows, arms, etc. It is one of the better methods of hair removal as there is no chance of razor burns, no ingrown hair, no cuts and very little chance of infection. Sometimes there may be red dots in the area of epilation, which last for a few hours and disappear on their own.

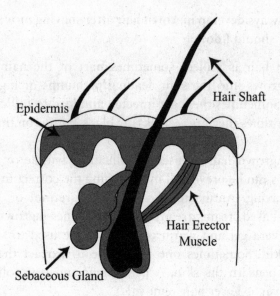

7. Is waxing a safe method for hair removal?

Yes, waxing is a safe and effective method for removing unwanted hair temporarily. Hair doesn't regrow fast, and the skin feels smooth after waxing. But one must take all the necessary precautions.

Do not wax sunburnt skin or very sensitive skin or if you have had a chemical peel or resurfacing Laser done within two weeks. Avoid using a retinol cream or exfoliating serum for at least five days before waxing. Always wash the area that needs to be waxed to remove all the dirt and grime before waxing. Use disposable cellophane strips for waxing, and never use wax that is more than a month old as it could be infected and cause boils. Make sure that the wax is properly stored, and hygiene is well maintained. After waxing, clean the area with lukewarm water and then apply a moisturizer on the skin.

8. Are there any side effects of waxing ?

Sometimes one may develop ingrown hair due to the pull on the hair follicle. If the wax was old or contaminated, or the wax strips and towels were not clean, one may develop folliculitis (bacterial infection of the hair follicle). Waxing may also be painful for some people.

9. I recently waxed my tummy and back. It was smooth for a few days, but then I developed a bad rash. It itches and hurts as well. I am worried that it will leave ugly marks. Please help. Also, the hair has grown back already. Should I avoid waxing again?

You must avoid waxing. Your hair follicles are prone to bacterial infection and rash due to the hair pull. Take a course of antibiotics and antiallergy medication for three days. Once the rash settles, apply a glycolic acid-based cream to get rid of the marks. You could try Laser hair removal. You may require six to eight sittings spaced six weeks apart depending on the density of the growth as well as the thickness of the hair.

10. Is it okay to pluck hair from the chin?

Plucking involves pulling of the hair, causing friction, which can result in post-inflammatory hyperpigmentation and sometimes scarring. Hence it is not advisable to pluck hair from any part of the face.

11. How can one get rid of white hair permanently?

While shaving, epilating, tweezing and waxing are temporary methods for removing white hair, the only permanent method so far is electrolysis. Laser does not work on white or grey hair because there is no melanin in white hair. Electrolysis can be a tedious and lengthy process because it involves inserting the electrode into each hair follicle and burning the follicle with an electrocautery device. Sometimes it may also cause burns or scars. So, it is better to go for Laser hair removal when the hair is naturally dark in colour.

12. What is dermaplaning?

Dermaplaning is a procedure that helps get rid of extremely fine hair, which is also known as peach fuzz. It is a finer form of shaving and uses a scalpel or a tool called the dermatome. It also helps exfoliate and remove dead skin, leaving the skin smooth, soft and clear.

There may be a little redness or soreness after dermaplaning so one must moisturize after the procedure. It must not be done if there is any active infection or inflammation such as herpes simplex infection, acne, rosacea, sunburn, eczema or psoriasis.

13. Is threading better than waxing the face?

Threading is an ancient hair removal technique usually done for small areas such as the eyebrows or even the face. A thread is used to tug the hair and pull it out with no chemicals used. Folliculitis or acne can occur due to threading. Sometimes, if the thread is infected, viral warts and molluscum contagiosum can spread from person to person due to threading. It is better to restrict this technique to the eyebrows and upper lip.

14. I get boils after waxing or shaving. Can I use a hair-removing cream?

Yes, using depilatory hair removal creams is a good option other than Laser hair removal. These creams contain thioglycolic acid, which breaks down the keratin in the hair and removes the hair by weakening the hair strands. They are safe to use provided one doesn't leave the cream on the skin for more than three to ten minutes, depending on the formulation. Always do a test patch behind the ear, i.e., apply a small quantity of the cream behind the ear, leave it on for three to ten minutes and then wipe it off. If there is any redness, irritation or burning, you should not use the depilatory cream. If there is no irritation or redness and the skin is clear and smooth, you can use the depilatory cream anywhere on the body. There are special mild creams made for the face and bikini area.

Do not use these creams if your skin is sunburnt or tanned, irritated or damaged or if you have recently had a chemical peel or fractional resurfacing treatment. You must also stop using AHA, BHA or retinol-based products for at least five days before using a depilatory cream. Should you have a burning sensation after applying the cream, wash it off immediately and apply a lot of ice. If the burning is severe, you may need to consult a dermatologist who will prescribe a cortisone cream. Always remember, if you leave the cream on the skin for too long, it can cause chemical burns and post-inflammatory hyperpigmentation.

15. How often can I bleach my hair, and is it safe to bleach?

Though not a dermatologist-recommended procedure, you may bleach your facial hair once in about three months provided your skin is not irritated or inflamed. Bleach contains hydrogen peroxide, which temporarily damages the pigment melanin, therefore making the hair look whiter or lighter. Sometimes bleach can cause an irritant reaction or a chemical burn. Hence it is important to do a test patch before bleaching. Never bleach within two weeks of any chemical or Laser treatment on the face. Make sure you always moisturize immediately after bleaching. Do not forget your sunscreen and do not step outdoors for at least twenty-four hours after bleaching.

16. Is Laser bleach a safer option than regular bleaching?

If you are allergic to bleaching creams or have had a reaction to bleaching in the past, it is better to opt for other methods of hair removal for fine hair or you can opt for Laser bleaching. Laser bleaching is a technique by which a Pico Laser or Q-switched Nd:YAG Laser is used with low fluence to destroy the melanin in the hair shaft thereby bleaching the hair without the use of a chemical. Indeed, it is a safe option, but you must make sure you do not step out in the sun for forty-eight hours after a Laser bleach procedure, especially to places like the beach or the hills.

LASER HAIR REMOVAL

Virtually your entire body is covered with hair. Because most of this hair is fine and pale, it usually isn't visible to the naked eye. But when darker, coarser hair appears in places that may make you uncomfortable—such as on the face, neck, abdomen, breasts, legs or underarms in women or on the shoulders, chest and back in men—it may be time to consider hair removal with a Laser.

1. What is Laser hair removal?

Hair removal, temporary or long term, has become an easier task with the advent of Lasers. Lasers that are safe and effective for use on Indian skin are: long-pulse alexandrite Laser, long-pulse diode Laser and long-pulse Nd:YAG Laser. The Laser light is absorbed by the hair follicle while other skin appendages are spared. Cooling devices attached to the Laser prevent heat damage to the surrounding skin. Laser hair removal needs multiple sessions. Hair regrowth is slower and scantier after each session.

2. Why should one opt for Laser hair reduction?

Laser hair reduction gets rid of unwanted facial and body hair. It is a wonderful alternative to the traditional methods of unwanted hair removal such as shaving, waxing, depilating and electrolysis.

3. Who can undergo Laser hair removal?

Anyone above the age of sixteen, both men and women, can have Laser hair reduction done to remove unwanted hair. Hair removal is commonly done on the underarms, pubic area, legs, upper lip, chin, back, buttocks, thighs, face, neck, chest, arms and toes.

4. How does a hair removal Laser work?

The Laser has a wavelength that specifically targets the pigment melanin contained in the hair follicle and shaft. The Laser pulses for a fraction of a second, penetrates the hair bulb without destroying the surrounding skin, and vaporizes the pigment in the hair follicle. Thus, the follicle is either destroyed or its regrowth impeded. This is a non-invasive procedure, and a large number of hairs are targeted in a single flash of light.

5. What precautions should I take before and after a Laser treatment?

Patients should not wax, epilate, bleach or pluck for at least four weeks prior to their first session and throughout the course of treatments.

6. How many Laser treatments does one need?

Most patients need at least eight to ten effective treatments spaced six to eight weeks apart. Because hair grows in cycles and the Laser targets only the hair in the anagen phase, several sessions are necessary to affect all hair in any given area. In case of a hormonal imbalance, one may need more sessions and maintenance sessions as well.

7. What are the causes of excessive hair growth?

The causes of excessive hair growth are many and varied, including heredity, pregnancy and hormonal imbalances (i.e., PCOS in women, insulin resistance, thyroid problems and reactions to certain medications).

Before starting Laser treatments, patients with excessive hair growth on uncommon areas should undergo investigations to explore possible underlying medical reasons for it. Hair removal methods can only impact hair that is currently growing. They cannot prevent the body from developing new hair due to underlying hormonal problems.

8. How much time does each session of Laser hair reduction take?

The time taken depends on the area of concern. The face usually takes about twenty minutes, both the underarms take about fifteen minutes and the legs could take about one to one-and a half hours and so on.

9. Are there any side effects of Laser hair reduction?

Usually there are no major side effects of Laser hair reduction other than minor redness and swelling just after the treatment, which can be resolved with the application of ice and cooling packs. There can be scab formation, which looks like a burn and will fall off in three to four days.

10. Is Laser hair reduction painful?

It is a pain-free procedure. Sometimes you may experience a sensation similar to a rubber band snapping against your skin, which lasts for about a second. In sensitive skin areas, we apply a numbing cream before the procedure to reduce the discomfort.

11. What precautions should I take before and after a Laser treatment?

You should use a sunscreen compulsorily. Do not apply any medicated creams for two to three days after the treatment. Do not wax, shave, epilate, bleach or pluck for at least six weeks prior to the Laser sessions or during the course of Laser treatments.

12. How long does it take for the hair to shed after Laser hair reduction?

Laser hair reduction is different from any other type of hair reduction. You will not notice hair reduction right away. Your hair will grow back after the session as it normally would, perhaps thinner and softer, and then ten to twelve days later it will start to shed.

13. What are the available Laser hair removal systems?

The most common Laser hair removal systems currently being used are long-pulse alexandrite Laser, long-pulse diode Laser, diode Laser with SHR technology, long-pulsed Nd: YAG Laser and intense pulse light or IPL.

14. Can Laser hair reduction help with ingrown hair?

Laser hair reduction is the only effective method for getting rid of ingrown hairs quickly. This is because Laser hair removal goes straight to the root or hair follicle. Once the follicle can no longer produce hair, the affected area heals.

If you do not have a hormonal imbalance, 95 to 98 per cent of the hair can be removed by Laser and the remaining

3 to 5 per cent are cosmetically acceptable. However, if you have a hormonal imbalance such as hyperandrogenism, PCOS, hypothyroidism, hyperprolactinemia, etc., the hair can grow back whenever there is an imbalance, so you will need maintenance sessions till the imbalance is treated. If you are taking oral steroid tablets or have been applying steroid creams for a long time, there are chances of new hair growth.

15. Does a long gap between Laser sessions make the treatment ineffective?

When you treat the hair with a Laser, all the hair in the anagen phase gets destroyed and does not grow back. So longer gaps between Laser sessions do not make the sessions ineffective. They just make the course of treatment very long because one needs about ten to twelve sessions at four to six weekly intervals.

16. Are triple wavelength Lasers better than single wavelength?

If the driver is good, he can drive any car well and take you to your destination. While triple wavelength Lasers may be 10 per cent faster and those who do not respond to conventional Lasers could try them as an alternative, single wavelength Lasers are equally effective and safe.

17. Why do men need Laser hair removal?

Men generally have hair on the ears (hypertrichosis), or they may have a unibrow or excessive hair on the upper parts of the cheeks. Sometimes they may be very hairy on the chest, back and arms. And some may frequently develop folliculitis or furunculosis in the hair-bearing areas. Hence, they seek options such as Laser hair removal. Other conditions such as hidradenitis suppurativa, which occurs typically in the underarms, or even pilonidal sinus, can be treated with Laser hair removal. In fact, Laser hair removal is a great option for all genders.

18. I always develop acne after a Laser hair removal session. What should I do to avoid this?

It is possible that your oil glands get triggered by the Laser or when shaving before the Laser treatment is performed. So, if you have a tendency to develop acne, you must inform your dermatologist, who will give you a short course of anti-acne medication whenever you have a Laser session.

19. Is there a chance of burns with Laser hair removal?

If the technician uses a very high energy or if you are sunburnt and you do a Laser hair removal procedure, there are chances of a burn. Hence, it is important to get the Laser procedure done from a reputed clinic, and to ensure that the technician performing the procedure is well qualified and well trained. Sometimes there may be mild scabbing or very superficial burns even if you get the procedure done at a reputed clinic because your skin is sensitive at the time of getting the treatment. In such a situation, it is best to apply ice and a mild cortisone cream and avoid sun exposure. This will help the scabs to dry and fall off without leaving any dark marks behind.

20. Can I bleach or wax between two sessions of Laser hair removal? Is Laser hair removal a lifetime treatment?

One should not bleach, wax, thread, pluck or tweeze hair between two Laser sessions. You can shave or trim between two Laser sessions. The idea is to keep the hair in the anagen phase with the roots intact so that the Laser can target the hair in the growing anagen phase during the next session.

21. Despite doing many Laser hair removal sessions, I continue to get new hair growth. What is the reason for this?

You either have a hormonal imbalance in the body or you need to change the type of Laser being used. Rarely, there are some non-responders too. So, consult with your dermatologist instead of repeatedly doing unsuccessful Laser sessions for your hair removal.

22. I am twenty-eight years old. I have excessive hair growth on my face. I went in for Laser hair removal on the upper lip, but that resulted in coarse regrowth and the upper lip area is now severely pigmented. It is embarrassing. Please suggest a remedy or a medicine that I can apply locally to remove the pigmentation. I do not want any more procedures.

It is unfortunate that you developed pigmentation after hair removal with a Laser. This may happen if the energy used is too high, causing epidermal burns. You may need to consult a dermatologist and use a cortisone cream once a day for a week to reduce the inflammation. Use vitamin

A and vitamin C serums to reduce the pigmentation. Avoid scrubbing and sun exposure. The best thing to do is to give it time to heal.

RAPID FIRE

1. Is Laser hair reduction safe for the reproductive system?

Laser hair reduction has no effect on fertility because the Laser has a specific wavelength that does not allow the energy to penetrate below the skin layers.

2. Is Laser hair reduction cancerous?

Laser hair reduction is absolutely non-cancerous.

3. Can I get Laser hair reduction done while I am pregnant?

Although Lasers have no effect on pregnancy, it is advisable to avoid getting the treatment done while you are pregnant.

4. Can white hair be removed with a Laser?

Unfortunately, white hair cannot be removed with a Laser because Laser can only destroy melanin, which is absent in white hair.

5. Is Laser hair removal painful?

The newer Lasers have an inbuilt cooling system that is far superior to the older devices. This numbs the skin, making the treatment virtually painless.

6. I am fifty-two years old. Can I opt for Laser hair removal or am I too old for it now?

There is no upper limit for Laser as far as age is concerned. As long as you have dark/black hair, you can opt for Laser hair removal. Remember, grey or white hair do not respond to Laser.

7. Is it possible to get rid of fine facial hair with Laser?

The long-pulse alexandrite Laser can be used to get rid of fine facial hair. However, if it is just peach fuzz, it is not advisable to use Laser.

8. Is it safe to do Laser hair removal if I have very dark skin?

Yes, the long-pulse alexandrite, the long-pulse diode and the long-pulse Nd Yag Lasers are safe for dark skin. The ruby Laser should not be used if the skin colour is dark.

9. Can Laser hair removal result in thin long hair growth?

Very rarely, if the Laser energy used to treat the hair is low, it may lead to paradoxical hair growth which appears as thin, long hair. But this could also be a result of a hormonal imbalance.

10. Can I Laser the hair over my tattoo?

You can, but your tattoo may disappear too!

15

Acne

'To heal a wound, you need to stop touching it.'
—Frank N. Stein

Acne is one of the top three dermatological problems encountered world over by teenagers as well as adults. It can be psychologically debilitating at times and requires attention. Greek physicians Aristotle and Hippocrates used the Greek words *ionthoi* and *varus* to describe acne as a condition that is strongly associated with puberty. In 1638, Riolanus associated acne in females with menstruation-related disorders. German physician Karl Gustav Theodor Simon was a hobbyist microscopist based in Berlin who, in 1842, saw a living, moving creature when examining tissue that was affected with acne. The term *acne vulgaris* (vulgaris

R. N. Grant. The History of Acne. *Proceedings of the Royal Society of Medicine.* 1951; 44; 647–652

means common) was first used by Fuchs in 1840 and has persisted to the present.

1. Are blackheads, pimples and acne different?

Blackheads, whiteheads and pimples are all different forms of acne. Mild to moderate acne is seen in the form of whiteheads (closed comedones). When whiteheads get exposed to light, they get oxidized and form blackheads. Then there are papules seen as tiny bumps on the skin, and pustules seen as pus-filled bumps (pimples). Severe acne is seen as nodules, cysts and abscesses, which lead to scarring if not treated in time. There can be truncal acne, i.e., acne on the chest and back or shoulders.

2. How does acne form?

Acne is a chronic inflammatory disorder of the sebaceous (oil) glands present in the skin.

During puberty or when there is a hormonal imbalance, the male sex hormones, which are normally present in both males and females, are on the rise, and they activate the sebaceous glands to increase in size, which in turn leads to an increase in the secretion of sebum. Second, cells are shed more rapidly and they stick together, plugging the opening of the hair follicle, resulting in 'whiteheads'. The pigment melanin in the whiteheads, when exposed to air, forms blackheads. Third, bacteria, especially cutibacterium acne, increases in number and results in pimples. When the follicle is clogged, its wall ruptures. The sebum, bacteria and dead cells escape into the surrounding tissue and lead to inflammation and formation of a more severe form of acne in the form of pustules, nodules, abscesses and cysts.

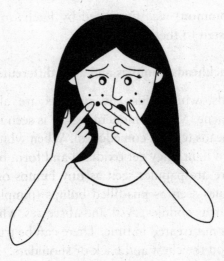

3. Isn't acne supposed to occur only in teenagers? Why do I have it when I'm thirty-eight?

Acne usually occurs due to a hormonal imbalance in the body or clogged, infected pores. It may start during puberty, but it can occur at any age. It is known as adult acne in the age group of thirty to fifty. In a study conducted in 2013 in Washington University, 43 per cent of individuals had acne in their thirties, 15–20 per cent females in their forties and fifties, and 7–12 per cent of males suffered from acne in their forties and fifties.

4. Is acne specific to women?

No, it occurs in both males and females. In fact, males have more sebaceous glands and higher sebaceous

Seattle WI. GBD Compare. Seattle: University of Washington; 2013.

gland activity. Thus, acne is actually more common in males.

5. Are there any don'ts if I have acne?

Yes, a poor lifestyle entailing an unhealthy diet (sugar, dairy, food with a high glycaemic index such as refined flour), late nights, alcohol, smoking, stress, comedogenic creams and body oils will aggravate acne. Gases from vehicle fuel as well as industrial gases can increase carbon monoxide, sulphur dioxide, nitrous oxide, volatile organic chemicals and fine particulate matter in the air, which in turn can clog pores, resulting in acne.

6. When should one opt for medical help?

The moment you see acne you should consult a dermatologist. Whether you take treatment or not is not the question, but you will at least know the dos and don'ts of acne and the right facewash, sunscreen and moisturizer to use. Your dermatologist will also help you find the cause of acne.

7. What are the causes of acne?

Acne usually occurs when the body goes through hormonal changes. Hence it is common during puberty in both males and females, and in females during periods, pregnancy and the perimenopausal phase as well. It can be genetic. It can also occur due to a hormonal imbalance as seen in polycystic ovary syndrome (PCOS), insulin resistance, hypothyroidism, hyperprolactinemia etc. Sometimes oil-based cosmetics, hair oils and brilliantines can clog pores and give rise to whiteheads, which can get infected and turn into pimples. People who work in chemical or oil industries and come in contact with hydrocarbons, heavy oils, cutting oil, wax, grease and coal tar derivatives, which can clog the pores, can develop acne. Drugs such as oral contraceptives, oral steroids, anabolic steroids, growth hormones, isoniazid, lithium, phenytoin, iodides, etc. can also cause acne.

8. I have acne-prone skin. What should my skincare routine be?

Use a facewash containing salicylic acid if you have whiteheads and blackheads. Salicylic acid will unclog pores and help reduce blackheads and whiteheads. You can also use facewashes containing grape seed extract, glycolic acid and tea tree oil to reduce the oiliness. You may opt for an alcohol-free toner after cleansing. However, it is not mandatory to use a toner. Use an oil-free, water- or gel-based moisturizer and water- or gel-based or matte sunscreen. Use a non-comedogenic make-up remover at bedtime. Do not use oil to remove make-up as oil can clog your pores and give you more acne. Follow it up with the cleanser, followed by a BHA, AHA or retinol serum on alternate nights. You may use a niacinamide-based serum on the other nights. If you are on medication for acne, after cleansing, use the medicated cream and follow it up with a moisturizer.

9. What home remedies can I try for acne?

You could try applying neem paste or pure aloe vera although I would personally advise you to consult with a dermatologist and avoid all home remedies. Do not apply lemon, toothpaste, apple cider vinegar or baking soda on pimples as this may result in post-inflammatory hyperpigmentation (PIH) and scarring.

10. Is there a particular diet I should follow if I have acne?

Drink about 2–3 litres of water unless you have a renal or heart condition and have been asked by your doctor to restrict your water intake. Have brightly coloured fruits and vegetables, which are rich in antioxidants (for example, berries, bell peppers, spinach, kale, etc.).

11. Should I be avoiding any food as I do break out into acne frequently?

Studies have shown that having food with a high glycaemic index such as fried potatoes and burgers, or sugar in any form (white sugar, jaggery, dates, coconut sugar) increases the insulin and insulin growth factor 1 (IGF-1) levels in the body, aggravating acne. Dairy products also increase the insulin and IGF-1 hormones. These will lead to increased androgen production, increased oil secretion and increased absorption of male hormones, all of which will result in acne.

12. When should one opt for medical help for acne? What kind of treatments are safe?

When acne persists in spite of using over-the-counter acne creams, or when you develop severe cystic or

F. Dall'Oglio, M. R. Nasca, F. Fiorentini, G. Micali. Diet and Acne: Review of the Evidence from 2009 to 2020. International Journal of Dermatology, June 2021; 60 (6): 672–685. doi: 10.1111/ijd.15390. Epub, 18 January 2021. PMID: 33462816.

nodular acne, or acne that leaves scars, you must seek medical help. In-clinic treatments such as carbon dioxide cryotherapy, plasma therapy, salicylic acid peels, mandelic acid peels, lactic acid peels and blue light therapy are safe to undergo.

13. Can I remove my blackheads and whiteheads at home? I have bought the clean-up instrument from Amazon.

Please do not try to do remove blackheads and whiteheads on your own. First, you may not be able to sterilize the clean-up instrument adequately and second, you may cause trauma to the deeper layers of the skin. This may lead to post-inflammatory hyperpigmentation or scarring. Do not pick or squeeze your acne either as this may lead to infection or damage to the deeper layers of the skin resulting in PIH and blemishes.

14. I have acne on my forehead and in the sidelocks area. Is it due to dandruff?

If you have dandruff due to a yeast infection called Malassezia furfur, the flakes can infect the skin along the hairline and cause bumps that look like acne. This has recently been called fungal acne by social media influencers. If you use hair products that contain ingredients that can clog your pores, you may get forehead and hairline acne. Avoid hair products used to smoothen the hair or products containing oils, petrolatum, mineral oil, acrylates, panthenol, silicone, quaternium-70, cyclopentasiloxane and dimethicone. If you need to use these products, you should rinse out the product and wash your scalp and hair thoroughly before going to bed.

15. Why do I get acne on my chest, back and shoulders?

Acne on the chest, back, shoulders and arms can occur due to various reasons. First, it could be genetic or hormonal. Oil massages on the body can clog the pores. Some hair products or hair oil on the scalp can trickle onto the body, leading to body acne. If you do not wash off your conditioner well, it may trickle onto your shoulders, chest and back, resulting in acne. Anabolic steroids, growth hormones and an excessive amount of protein powders containing casein can also result in body acne. Friction due to backpacks, excessive sweating, etc., are other causes of body acne.

16. I am a nineteen-year-old guy. I eat healthy, sleep well, exercise and take care of my skin and still get pimples.

At nineteen, you are developing acne due to hormonal changes occurring in your body. Please continue to eat healthy, avoid sugar, dairy and food with a high glycaemic index. Follow your circadian rhythm and sleep early. Make sure you learn to cope with stress; stress can play a major role in aggravating acne. Consult with a dermatologist for proper guidance.

17. I get acne only on one side of my face. Why?

You could either be sleeping on one side such that the dust from your pillow cover is clogging your pores. Or you could be holding your cell phone too close to the skin, and that side of the cheek could develop acne both due to friction or dirt on your cell phone. If you have hair falling on one side of your face, the sebum or products in your hair can clog pores and cause acne.

Sometimes one may have more oil glands on one side of the face than the other.

If possible, use silk or satin pillow covers. Change the pillow covers every two days. Keep your cell phone clean; alternatively, use ear pods. Keep your hair away from your face. Avoid touching your face with dirty fingers.

18. I have to wear make-up every day as I am a flight attendant. I am twenty-one years old. I had acne as a teenager, so I am worried I will get it again. What sort of make-up should I opt for?

First of all, follow a good skincare routine of cleansing, moisturizing and using a sunscreen in the day. Remove your make-up at night and use a salicyclic acid serum thrice a week at bedtime. As for make-up, opt for water-based, oil-free make-up. Liquid foundations are better than creams and mousse. Look for labels like hypoallergenic and non-comedogenic, oil-free and 'won't clog pores'. The foundations and concealers you use should not contain ingredients such as oils, wax, paraffin, petrolatum, lanolin, etc., which can occlude your pores, resulting in inflammation and acne. Opt for lighter formulations as and when possible. Do not forget to double cleanse and remove all your make-up at bedtime. Make sure your make-up brushes, beauty blenders and sponges are clean. You must wash them once every week and store them in a clean place. Do not share your make-up applicators or make-up with anyone.

19. My pimples improve when I am on medication, but I break out again a few months after I stop taking the medication.

You need to make lifestyle changes. Stop having food with sugar, dairy, refined flour and fried potatoes. Avoid applying comedogenic products. Follow a skincare routine meant for acne-prone skin. Do not try all the new serums and products advertised on social media. Get your hormones checked; you may be suffering from PCOS, hyperthyroidism or insulin resistance.

20. My dermatologist prescribed antibiotics for me because I have large pimples on my face. I always thought antibiotics cause acne. Please clarify.

Bacteria called Cutibacterium acne (C. acne) are the major occupant of the pilosebaceous unit (the hair and oil glands in the skin together form a unit called the pilosebaceous unit). Accounting for up to 90 per cent of the microbiota in sebum-rich sites such as the scalp, face, chest and back, C. acne gradually increases from puberty to adulthood and then decreases after the age of fifty. When there is an overload of C. acne, blackheads or whiteheads can turn into pus-filled pimples. Thus, specific antibiotics against C. acne are prescribed as per US Food and Drug Administration (FDA) regulations.

21. My doctor has prescribed isotretinoin. I am scared to take it as I have heard it has side effects.

Isotretinoin is a derivative of vitamin A. It is a well-researched, US FDA-approved molecule and can be taken under medical supervision. Ten to 40 milligrams of isotretinoin can be taken safely depending on the body weight. It may cause dryness and chapped lips, but one can use a moisturizer and lip balm to combat the dryness.

Isotretinoin has teratogenic effects on the foetus. Hence it is not safe to take during pregnancy. The last traces of isotretinoin are said to get flushed from the body a month after consuming the last dose. It is better to stop using isotretinoin three months before one plans to conceive. The liver and cholesterol levels should be checked every three months. If there is a genetic predisposition to hyperlipidemia or if a person has raised cholesterol or is taking an antidepressant, isotretinoin should be avoided.

22. I have a twelve-year-old who is beginning to get pimples. Should this be treated or left as a normal process of puberty?

The moment pimples occur, you should consult with a dermatologist to begin proper skincare and at least some form of topical application to control the acne. Please do not leave it as a normal process of puberty as there may be a possibility of severe acne and scarring in the days to come. Acne is neither normal nor curable. It can be controlled with the help of medicines, a proper skincare routine and a healthy lifestyle.

23. I get dark marks after every pimple heals. I have a lot of blemishes. What can I do?

First of all, do not squeeze your pimples and don't try any home remedies. Both could lead to post-inflammatory hyperpigmentation. Protect your skin from UV rays and blue light by applying an oil-free sunscreen. Take supplements of vitamin C. Avoid excessive scrubbing or exfoliation. Sometimes the body has a tendency to hyperpigment during the healing process, be it a cut, wound or pimple. Use pigment-lightening creams that do not contain steroids, hydroquinone or comedogenic agents. A few sessions of chemical peels such as glycolic acid, salicylic acid, mandelic acid or TCA done strictly at skin clinics will help get rid of the blemishes.

24. My pimple dries when I apply toothpaste but it always leaves a black mark. What should I do?

Toothpaste may contain baking soda, triclosan and synthetic compounds that can dry out a pimple. But these ingredients can also irritate the skin and cause post-inflammatory hyperpigmentation which may takes many months to go or may even lead to scars. Avoid using toothpaste on your pimple and consult a dermatologist. You may also follow the tips given in the previous answer.

25. Can constipation cause pimples?

There is no study showing a direct correlation between acne and constipation. However, if there is an overload of microorganisms in the intestines due to constipation and the intestinal barrier is disrupted, the gut microbes enter the bloodstream, reach the skin and disturb the skin equilibrium. This may result in acne.

26. Is there any correlation between the gut and acne?

When one suffers from stress, anxiety, depression or is constantly worried, the brain sends signals to the gut resulting in inflammation of the intestines and leading to a disruption in the intestinal barrier. Gut microbes and their neurotransmitters (i.e., acetylcholine, serotonin, norepinephrine) cross the intestinal mucosa to enter the bloodstream and result in systemic inflammation and acne.

27. Will consuming probiotics improve my acne?

Yes, probiotics will improve acne especially if acne is associated with stress or gut infections.

Stress impairs the normal gut microflora, especially the Lactobacillus and Bifidobacterium species. This can result in an increase of certain microbes in the skin such as Cutibacterium acnes, Malassezia furfur, etc. Probiotics can suppress Cutibacterium acnes through the secretion of antibacterial protein. Probiotics may also lower the glycaemic load, reduce IGF-1 signalling and ultimately decrease proliferation of skin cells called keratinocytes as well as overactivity of sebaceous glands.

28. After every clean-up in a parlour, I get more pimples. Why does this happen?

While removing blackheads or whiteheads, if a portion of the sebum plug remains behind, it can lead to inflammation and pimples. Thus, the person doing the extractions should make sure the entire comedone is extracted. Second, if the instrument used for the extraction of blackheads and whiteheads is not sterile, it may lead to inflammation or a secondary bacterial infection.

Lee YB, Byun EJ, Kim HS. Potential Role of the Microbiome in Acne: A Comprehensive Review. J Clin Med. 2019;8(7):987. Published 2019 Jul 7. doi:10.3390/jcm8070987

(Salem I, Ramser A, Isham N, Ghannoum MA. The Gut Microbiome as a Major Regulator of the Gut-Skin Axis. Front Microbiol. 2018;9:1459. Published 2018 Jul 10. doi:10.3389/fmicb.2018.01459)

29. I'm fed up of blackheads on my nose. Is there any permanent solution?

Blackheads on the nose or anywhere on the face can occur due to sebum production by the sebaceous glands present on the nose. There may not be a permanent cure, but you can surely reduce them by applying a cream such as 2.5 per cent benzoyl peroxide or adapalene gel as prescribed by your dermatologist. Use a facewash containing salicylic acid. Chemical exfoliation with AHA or BHA serums can reduce blackheads. If you have oily skin, leave the serum on overnight, but if you have dry skin, leave it on for about two to three hours and remove it and wash your face. Salicylic acid is a good exfoliant, and it helps remove the excess skin cells on the surface of the pore so they don't build up in the pore. Use blackhead removal strips occasionally. You could get the blackheads removed once a month at a cosmetic clinic. You could also get a microdermabrasion done once a month. Sometimes hair on the nose can increase blackheads. So, Laser hair removal from the nose would help. You can also try the following home remedy: Take one teaspoon

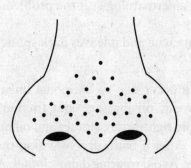

of red lentils (masoor dal) and one teaspoon of raw rice and powder coarsely. Add half a teaspoon of honey to it. Make a paste and use this as a scrub. Gently scrub your nose and rinse with lukewarm water. Warm water will remove the oil and the coarse powder will unclog your pores. This is called mechanical exfoliation. Do not scrub vigorously. Vigorous scrubbing can lead to post-inflammatory hyperpigmentation.

30. What is maskne? How can I prevent it?

Wearing a mask covers the face due to which the pores can get clogged with sweat and sebum and with creams or cosmetics that one applies. This will result in whiteheads or pus-filled acne called maskne. Wear a clean disposable mask. When you want to remove the mask while eating, keep it in a clean place upside down. If you wear cloth masks, make sure you wash them every day with a fragrance-free detergent. Make sure you cleanse your face well before wearing a mask. Apply a water- or gel-based or lightweight moisturizer. Avoid thick creams, oils and make-up under the mask. At bedtime, you can double cleanse and use a BHA serum to reduce the maskne. Please consult with a dermatologist if the problem persists.

31. I have butt acne and it leaves dark spots. What should I do?

Butt acne can occur due to hormonal imbalance, insulin resistance, sweat, oil massage and friction due to tight clothing. Avoid tight-fitting clothes and oil massages. Keep yourself dry. After a bath, dry your skin thoroughly and apply powder. Avoid wearing damp clothes. Any hormonal imbalance needs to be treated. At night, apply an anti-acne cream prescribed by a dermatologist. Chemical peels help in getting rid of the dark spots.

32. Is there such a thing as 'seasonal acne', which happens because of the change of season?

The effect of seasons on acne is variable. Some people experience worsening of their acne in winters while others in summer. Rise in temperature, increased humidity and sweating are the reasons why acne can be aggravated in summer. In winter, dryness causes the body to produce more sebum, causing clogged pores and hence breakouts.

33. What are the signs and symptoms of PCOS?

Polycystic ovary syndrome (PCOS) is called a syndrome as it is a combination of various signs and symptoms in the body such as acne, alopecia (hair loss), hirsutism (hair growth on face and body), acanthosis nigricans (thick, velvety dark discoloration of body folds and neck), obesity and irregular menstrual cycles. Raised androgen (male hormones) levels, raised insulin levels due to insulin resistance or the appearance of tiny cysts in the ovaries detected on ultrasonography are commonly seen. Insulin resistance is one of the main reasons behind skin manifestations of PCOS. When the cells in your muscles, fat and liver do not respond well to the existing insulin hormone in your body, they cannot use glucose from your blood for energy. As a result, the pancreas tries to compensate by producing more insulin, resulting in raised sugar levels over time. Some patients with normal weight can have lean PCOS. A person suffering from PCOS need not necessarily have all the signs and symptoms of PCOS.

34. Is acne due to PCOS a common thing?

When I started practising way back in 2000, I would see acne mostly in teenagers. Now, I see more and more adults in their late thirties and forties with acne. Two decades ago, I would come across two to three cases of PCOS associated acne in a week. Now I see three to four cases per day! Unhealthy lifestyle comprising unhealthy diet, late nights, alcohol, smoking and stress are the reasons for this rise in acne. Gases from vehicle fuel as well as industrial gases can increase carbon monoxide, sulphur dioxide, nitrous oxide, volatile organic chemicals and fine particulate matter in the air which in turn can clog pores, resulting in acne both in teenagers as well as adults.

35. How does one manage PCOS?

Diet and lifestyle modifications are among the first-line treatments for PCOS. Acne, hair fall, acanthosis and even hormone levels resolve by a great degree just by changing one's lifestyle. Weight loss of up to 5 to 10 per cent of the body weight will improve symptoms of PCOS.

High-fibre foods with low glycaemic index such as green leaves, seeds and whole grains act as antioxidants, which fight to lower inflammation, improve gut bacteria and lower insulin levels. Lean protein in the form of fish, skinless chicken and plant protein sources will help in weight loss, which in turn decreases androgen levels responsible for hirsutism, cystic acne or even irregular menstrual cycles. Sugar in any form and refined flour should be strictly avoided. These are great for the palate but increase insulin resistance. Alcohol can cause zinc deficiency, inflammation and fatty liver, all indirectly leading to an imbalance in hormones, triggering the symptoms of PCOS. Smoking increases free testosterone and is detrimental to those with PCOS.

In adults and adolescents with PCOS, strict physical activity sessions for at least thirty minutes a day or 150 minutes a week are recommended. This will help in weight loss and will also help maintain a BMI of less than 24. A raised BMI does not allow insulin levels to come down, resulting in persistence of the symptoms of PCOS. Stress can aggravate your cortisol hormones, which in turn will increase insulin resistance. It would be a good idea to engage in meditation, yoga or anything that helps you cope with stress. Disturbed sleep as well as late nights will alter the cortisol levels and are equally bad. A healthier lifestyle and weight loss will also reduce the long-term risks for diabetes, abnormal triglyceride levels, hypertension and cardiovascular disease in patients of PCOS.

In addition to lifestyle modifications, consuming supplements of vitamin B6, folic acid, inositol, chromium, selenium, magnesium, zinc, alpha lipoic acid, carnitine and omega 3 fatty acids has beneficial effects. Studies have also shown that low vitamin B12, vitamin D3 and calcium can increase insulin resistance. So, it is imperative that the blood levels be checked and the vitamins replenished if low. In severe cases of PCOS, oral contraceptives, flutamide, etc. are prescribed as standard FDA-approved drugs and can be safely taken under the supervision of a gynaecologist or endocrinologist. Metformin is a wonder drug in cases of insulin resistance.

In those suffering from acne, anti-acne creams containing clindamycin, benzoyl peroxide, retinol or azelaic acid are prescribed along with systemic minocycline or lymecycline. Chemical peels or blue light therapy also help reduce inflammation and blemishes. In cases of hirsutism, Laser hair removal with a long-pulsed diode Laser, alexandrite Laser or a long-pulsed Nd Yag Laser is safe and effective. However, one must lose weight and improve one's lifestyle before going ahead with the Laser hair removal sessions. In those with hair fall, the supplements mentioned above help bring the hair back to the growing anagen cycle from the telogen cycle. It is better to avoid heat and chemical treatments to the hair when there is excessive hair shedding. Stress should be kept at bay to prevent hair fall as well as acne. For acanthosis, metformin and weight loss are the only solution.

All in all, studies have shown that by merely following a healthy lifestyle and diet, PCOS can be easily controlled.

36. What skincare routine should be followed for acne during pregnancy?

It is best to avoid salicylic acid in your facewashes or serums. Use a facewash containing tea tree oil or grape seed extract or even glycolic acid to reduce oiliness. Azelaic acid in serums or gels can be used to reduce acne. Benzoyl peroxide, clindamycin and erythromycin can be used in moderation as per your dermatologist's advice. Oral isotretinoin or topical tretinoin, tazarotene, retinol, adapalene or any other retinol and its derivatives are strictly prohibited during pregnancy. Oral doxycycline, minocycline and lymecycline should not be consumed.

You may get clean-ups and AHA peels at a skin clinic, but avoid salicylic acid peels and Laser treatments.

37. All my PCOS reports are normal, but I still get acne and my dermatologist says it is due to PCOS. Please help.

If you have any two out of three criteria positive (irregular periods or symptoms such as acne, hair loss, hirsutism or abnormal blood levels), you can have PCOS even if your reports are normal. Hence follow the instructions given by your dermatologist. Make sure you lead a healthy lifestyle and maintain a BMI of 25 or less.

38. I only get acne before my period. How do I prevent or treat this?

This is purely hormonal since the oestrogen and progesterone levels drop just before menstrual cycles. Avoid eating sugar, milk, potatoes and refined flour during this period. Avoid using any comedogenic products on the face. Apply a BHA serum on the entire face on alternate nights as a preventive measure. BHA or salicylic acid is a good option to unclog pores and reduce oil. Your dermatologist may give you oral medication in severe cases.

39. I never had acne in my teens. I am forty-five now, and I have acne along my jawline.

Adult acne can occur at any age. It is usually seen around the chin and jawline. Most of the times, it is a result of a hormonal imbalance in the body, especially in females. The imbalance can occur around periods, pregnancy, perimenopause and menopause, or after discontinuing (or starting) birth control pills. An imbalance can also occur as a result of stress, use of oil-based comedogenic products or facial massages especially with oils, which can clog the pores. The skincare routine is the same as for those with acne-prone skin as discussed earlier. Your dermatologist may prescribe isotretinoin, oral contraceptives, finasteride, Aldactone, flutamide or metformin, depending on the need. Do not use oil-based products on the face and scalp.

40. What is acne mapping?

Face mapping originated in China. Acne face mapping divides sections of the face and relates certain areas to organs that cause pimples to arise there. However, acne can occur all over the face and face mapping does not always hold true.

Acne on the forehead could be due to hair oils or comedogenic hair products. Whiteheads and blackheads on any one side of the cheek could be due to dirty pillowcases or cell phone covers. Chin and jawline acne is usually hormonal. Acne in the T-zone occurs in those with combination skin.

41. Can tea tree oil be used in the treatment of acne?

Tea tree oil is derived from the Melaleuca alternifolia tree, which is native to Australia. The oil contains several antimicrobial substances, and a study showed that formulations with a 5 per cent tea tree oil concentration help reduce acne without causing any irritation. However, over-the-counter tea tree oil formulations have a concentration of only 1 per cent.

Daily habits to prevent acne

1. Before you hit the bed, be sure to remove your make-up and clean your face no matter how tired you may be. Make-up along with the entire day's dust, sweat salts, soot and grime can clog pores and result in zits or even an itchy rash.
2. Clean your cell phone cover. You may be keeping your phone in various places through the day and the phone accumulates dust and bacteria on the cover. This will infect the side of the face that comes in contact with the phone when you use it.
3. Change your pillow covers thrice a week. You may be washing your face regularly but if your pillow covers haven't been changed in three days, you can be sure they are laden with bacteria and dust mites, which can result in whiteheads, pustules, rashes or just an itchy face.
4. Do not touch your face. Our hands are full of microorganisms, billions of them at any given time. They get transferred to your face when you pop a zit or keep touching your face. And you never know when one of these microorganisms will turn wicked and cause boils or pus-filled acne on your face.
5. Change your cosmetics. If your foundation, concealer, blush, lipstick or eye make-up are older than a year, you need to throw them out. Also, make sure you always check the expiry date of your moisturizers, day and night creams.

> 6. Wash your make-up sponges and brushes at least twice a week. Imagine the dust and germs sitting on your brushes, which you then use on your face. You are sure to get allergies, whiteheads or painful zits.
>
> 7. Wash your hands before digging into those jars with creams. It is better to use a clean spatula instead.

RAPID FIRE

1. I drink a lot of water, so why do I still get acne?

Acne occurs due to hormonal imbalance or prodcucts which clog your pores. While water is important to maintain your skin hydration, it doesn't play a role in clearing acne.

2. I am thirteen years old and have acne. But I am told that it is normal to have acne and they will go on their own. Is it true?

While it is completely normal to have acne at the age of thirteen, it is important to consult a dermatologist and treat the acne. You may develop scars if you don't treat acne on time.

3. Can blood purifiers clear my acne?

Scientifically, there is nothing like impure blood and blood purifiers have no role to play in the treatment of acne.

4. Do people with a lot of heat in the body get more acne?

Fever, infections and exercise can increase the body temperature but will not cause acne.

5. Can lack of hygiene and dirt on the face cause acne?

Dirt can clog pores and result in folliculitis or mila. Bad skin hygiene can result in bacteria entering the existing blackheads and whiteheads and cause pus-filled pimples.

6. Is it important to get facials regularly to prevent acne?

Facials include massaging the skin with oils and creams. Massage itself will stimulate the oil glands to produce more oil triggering more acne formation. So instead of facials, opt for clean ups at skin clinics whenever required.

7. I have taken medicines for acne for two weeks but there is no improvement. Should I change my doctor?

It takes at least six to eight weeks for acne to come under control. So please give it time. Changing the doctor wont help.

8. Will my acne improve if I scrub my skin daily?

No, on the contrary, frequent scrubbing may damage your skin and lead to more acne.

9. Are blackheads caused due to dirt?

No, when your pores clogged with excess oil and dead cells is exposed to air, they gets oxidized and turn black.

10. Should I pop my pimple to make it go away quickly?

Not only do you run the risk of developing an infection when you pop a zit, you may also develop post-inflammatory hyperpigmentation which looks like black marks or even scarring. So do not pop pimples.

16

Skin Texture

'Nature gives you the face you have at twenty; it is up to you to merit the face you have at fifty.'
—Coco Chanel

The texture of the skin is defined by the smoothness on its surface. When there are irregularities on the skin's surface due to bumps, acne, acne scars, warts, skin tags, moles, dryness and accumulation of dead skin, light which falls on the skin doesn't get reflected. This leads to the appearance of dull skin and rough texture. There are various methods to improve our skin texture, from chemical exfoliation with AHA, BHA or retinoids to treatments like microneedling, fractional Lasers, etc.

Acne scars are one of the commonest reasons for uneven texture as well as a youngster's low self-esteem. Some of the common skin texture issues have been discussed here.

ACNE SCARS

1. What are acne scars?

Scars which are seen as a result of acne are known as acne scars. Blemishes are the most common and are seen as dark spots when a pimple or a blackhead or whitehead subsides. Pits or depressions on the skin surface are seen in various shapes and sizes. In medical terminology, they are known as depressed atrophic scars and are classified as rolling or box or ice pick scars. The third type of scars, tiny, raised skin-coloured bumps known as popular scars, are commonly seen on the nose and chin. The fourth type are known as keloidal scars. They are raised, irregular, large and reddish is colour.

2. How are acne scars formed?

When large pimples or acne are left untreated, they may heal with a pit or a depression or what is known as a scar due to severe inflammation. The second reason for scars is self-picking or bursting blackheads, whiteheads, pustules and pimples. These will result in blemishes and pits. Use of garlic, lime, lemon and other such acidic ingredients or scrubbing too much can also result in blemishes or scarring.

3. Can I use any creams to get rid of my acne scars?

For mild scars, one may use a retinol- or glycolic acid-based product on alternate nights. Avoid using too much product and avoid daily use as it may cause irritation and severe scaling. For blemishes, one may use products with

vitamin C, kojic acid, arbutin, lactic acid, mandelic acid
or salicylic acid in them.

4. Are there any general skincare habits that one must follow to avoid scars from forming?

Most certainly! One must not pick at the acne. That one
pimple on your face may be difficult to resist but pop it
and you will end up with an ugly scar, which can take
up to two years to go on its own. Second, touching or
popping your zits will result in bacterial infection and
pus formation.

Scrubbing or exfoliating too much will also disrupt
the protective layer of the skin, causing more damage and
pigmentation. Not cleansing your face at bedtime and not
removing make-up before you sleep will also clog pores,
resulting in more acne and acne scars. Get a clean-up at a
skin clinic once in a month if you get regular breakouts or
blackheads. This will prevent the formation of deep scars.
However, this can be a catch-22 situation. If the clean-up
is not done correctly, you may end up with scars too.

5. My sister and I both have acne. But her face doesn't scar and mine scars terribly. Why is that so?

If you have very high levels of androgens or PCOS,
you are likely to scar more. Besides, every skin type is
different. Some scar easily, some don't. Make sure you
don't pick at your acne and always use sunscreen during
the day. Do not try home remedies such as using lemon,
toothpaste, garlic paste, baking soda, etc. as they may
cause more harm than good to your skin.

6. I have a lot of blemishes caused by acne. They do not seem to go with any creams. What can I do?

If they are old or do not improve with creams, one may go for glycolic acid, mandelic acid, tretinoin or TCA peels. These peels are done once in a fortnight and about eight to twelve sessions are required to get rid of blemishes. Read the chapter on peels for more details.

7. I have a lot of acne scars, which look like craters on my face, and I am losing my confidence due to them. What can I do? Will my skin ever be smooth again?

Acne scars can be treated with a variety of combination treatments depending on the depth and type of scars. Ice-pick scars are treated with cross TCA peels and fractional Lasers. Rolling and box scars are treated with radio frequency microneedling and fractional Lasers. Subcision may be done for all types of scars. If the pits are mild, microneedling with Dermapen helps on young skin. In those above thirty years, radio frequency microneedling is a better option as radio frequency helps to tighten the skin too. For deep pits, one has to do a combination of subcision, fractional Lasers like ResurFX, radio frequency microneedling and peels. Your dermatologist will plan the treatments at monthly intervals, and it can take one to one-and-a-half years for a significant amount of improvement in the acne scars. Make sure you go to a qualified dermatologist for all of the above treatments.

8. I have acne scars on my face and have read about Lasers, microneedling and platelet-rich plasma therapy. Which option is 100 per cent effective?

First of all, no treatment is 100 per cent effective and second, the type and depth of scars vary in every individual. Usually one has a combination of ice pick scars, rolling scars and box scars and sometimes they may be hypertrophic scars. Hence one treatment modality will never work. One usually has to opt for a combination of all of the above treatments depending on the type and depth of scars. Remember, it takes up to a year or more to see an improvement with all these treatments. It is not overnight magic.

9. I have read that fractional Laser treatment will reduce my acne scars and pores. I am forty years old. Should I be going for it or is it too late?

You can certainly go for a fractional Laser treatment although it would have been better if you had treated your acne scars within a year of their appearance. There is no age bar for fractional Laser treatment. You can do it from the age of eighteen to eighty if you have acne scars, fine lines, open pores, stretch marks, chicken pox scars, post-injury scars, stitch marks and even just for skin tightening.

Both Fractional CO_2 or Erbium Lasers may be used and give good results. Most of them such as the Resurfx, which we use at Skinfinitii, are US FDA-approved for skin resurfacing. The Resurfx device works on Laser energy to create multiple microscopic injuries over the treated area. These minuscule injuries release multiple growth factors, which causes new collagen formation along with the remodelling of existing collagen. As the collagen remodels, the fine lines and pores improve and the crinkled skin over the face and neck tightens, giving an anti-aging effect. There is redness and swelling on the face for about forty-eight hours after treatment. One should strictly avoid sun exposure after a Laser treatment for at least a week to prevent post-inflammatory hyperpigmentation.

10. I am getting married in four months. I have some acne pits and blemishes on my face. I want to get rid of them before my wedding. Please tell me the best treatment options.

Since you have only four months left for your wedding, it is better to get glycolic acid and TCA peels done to get rid of the blemishes. This will take about three months. You could also do two sessions of platelet-rich plasma therapy and microneedling with Dermapen in addition to the peels to reduce the depth of the pits.

These are safe treatments, but stop them fifteen days before your wedding. If you have wider scars and you want a quick fix, you may opt for hyaluronic acid filler injections.

11. My daughter is eighteen years old. She had chicken pox two years ago. It left a lot of scars on her face and neck. Can you please tell me what medication can help get rid of the scars?

Pitted facial scars caused by chicken pox respond poorly to topically applied medication such as retinoic acid,

AHAs, etc. She will need to undergo a combination of fractional Laser, platelet-rich plasma therapy and radio frequency microneedling. The combination is effective and safe and can give a 60 to 70 per cent improvement in scars. For a quick fix, you can opt for hyaluronic acid filler injections.

Please remember that there are very effective antiviral therapies for chicken pox these days. So, please do not go by the old myth of 'it will go by itself'. Oral antiviral drugs like acyclovir significantly shorten the duration and magnitude of the disease, accelerate healing, reduce the number of skin lesions and reduce the chances of scarring in healthy young individuals.

SKIN TAGS

1. What are skin tags?

Skin tags, or acrochordons, occur as tiny skin-coloured growths most commonly on the neck, the underarms and sometimes on the face, thighs or any other part of the body. When they are flat, they are called dermatosis papulose nigra and may be seen on the face, neck, chest, abdomen, back and arms. People often confuse them with warts. Skin tags are not the result of an infection, unlike warts, which are of viral origin.

2. Why does one develop skin tags?

Skin tags are either genetic or occur due to friction in body folds in those who are overweight. They are also prevalent in people who are pre-diabetic, or suffering from diabetes, insulin resistance, PCOS and metabolic syndrome. They have also been seen to occur during pregnancy. Some studies have found that if one has higher levels of insulin growth factor (IGF-1) and more insulin growth factor receptors, they are more likely to develop skin tags.

3. How do I prevent skin tags?

If the causes are genetic or pregnancy, you cannot prevent skin tags. But if you are obese or have a metabolic disorder, it is advisable to lose weight and maintain your BMI below 25.

4. Can I use dental floss or garlic juice to remove my skin tag?

I have seen people use various kinds of home remedies and end up with an infection, post-inflammatory hyperpigmentation or even scarring. Please do not use dental floss, apple cider vinegar, garlic juice, caustic lime or even horse hair to remove your skin tags. Please get them removed at a skin clinic by a doctor.

5. How can skin tags be removed?

Skin tags are usually cauterized using radio frequency or CO_2 Laser. If the tag is slightly large in size, it can be removed surgically. All these procedures are safe, in-clinic procedures and have minimal downtime.

6. Will skin tags grow back after being removed?

Skin tags do not grow back after removal. However, you may develop new ones in other areas of the body.

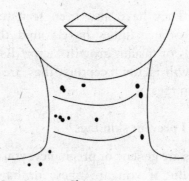

Skin tags

7. Can skin tags be cancerous?

No, skin tags are never pre-malignant or cancerous.

8. Are skin tags the same as warts?

Skin tags are often labelled as warts. However, warts usually have a cauliflower shape or rough skin surface. They are contagious and are of viral origin, typically human papilloma virus. Warts should be cauterized or treated with liquid nitrogen cryotherapy. Warts can regrow in spite of removing them once.

MOLES

1. Why do moles appear and can they appear at any age?

Moles are either genetic or can occur due to excessive sun exposure. They usually occur during childhood and can change in colour and size as one grows. Sometimes new moles appear in adults when the hormones change. They could also occur during pregnancy.

2. Can moles be removed?

If the moles are fairly large and can be felt with the fingers, they can be excised surgically or with a Laser. Flat moles can be removed with a Q-switched Nd:YAG or Pico Lasers.

3. When should one worry about a mole?

If a mole changes shape, texture or colour or if it grows rapidly within six weeks, one should get it tested by a dermatologist. Some melanocytic nevi can be pre-cancerous.

4. I am a thirty-seven-year-old woman and over the last five to seven years I have started developing red moles all over my body. They are not painful or itchy, but I want to know whether they could be dangerous.

These red moles are known as cherry angiomas. They are benign skin growths made up of blood vessels. They are genetic and harmless. Sometimes they occur due to aging and sometimes they are even seen during pregnancy. If you want to get them removed due to cosmetic reasons, you could opt for removal with radio frequency

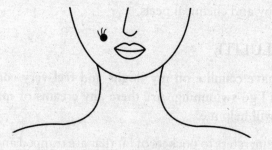

Mole on face

cautery, cryotherapy or Laser. If they don't bother you cosmetically, you can let them be.

PORES

1. I have very large, open pores. Is there a way to close them?

Pores do not have windows or doors that will open and close. They are normal openings of sebaceous glands on the surface of the skin, and there are approximately 20,000 pores on the face itself. Hence it is not possible to close pores. However, if there is excessive oil secretion, the pore, which is the opening of the duct leading to the oil glands, can get clogged and subsequently enlarged. Chemical exfoliants such as salicylic acid can help unclog these pores. Retinol and alpha hydroxy acid-based serums can also help reduce pore size at a younger age. Pores are held intact by collagen fibres. With age, these fibres degrade and the support to the duct as well as the opening reduces, thereby resulting in enlarged pores. While retinol serums may show minimal improvement, pore size can only be reduced with treatments such as radio frequency microneedling, fractional Lasers, platelet-rich plasma therapy and chemical peels.

CELLULITE

1. I have cellulite on my thighs and feel very conscious when I go swimming. Are there any creams or massages that will help me?

Cellulite refers to pockets of fat that are trapped and cause dimpling in the skin. This dimpling is irregular and patchy and has been likened to an orange peel. It gets aggravated by a sedentary lifestyle, crash diets, less water intake, diet pills, sleeping pills, alcohol, caffeine and smoking. So, one must avoid all these factors to improve the appearance of the areas of cellulite. However, no creams or exercise can reduce cellulite. Subcision, endermologie, Laser, acoustic wave therapy and Cellfina are some of the treatment options that give about 50 to 60 per cent results. The latest US FDA-approved treatment is in the form of injections called QWO.

STRETCH MARKS

1. I have stretch marks on my arms and shoulders. Is there any way to get rid of them?

Stretch marks are the result of the rapid stretching of the skin due to weight gain, pregnancy or when there is rapid muscle growth due to exercise. If the stretch marks are less than six months old or if they are violet or pink in colour, they can be treated with the application of tretinoin 0.025 per cent and silicon-based gel for a few months. If the marks are white in colour and old, it may not be possible to get rid of them completely. A combination of radio frequency microneedling, fractional Lasers and platelet-rich plasma treatment will help reduce the stretch marks.

2. I am planning a baby soon. Are there are any preventive measures I can take to avoid stretch marks?

Stretch marks occur due to rapid stretching of the elastin fibres in the skin. You cannot prevent them from occurring during pregnancy. But you can reduce the intensity by applying a mix of oils such as coconut oil, almond oil and bio oil two to three times a day. Massage the abdomen gently after applying the oil. Make sure you have a healthy diet, exercise routinely and do not gain unnecessary weight.

RAPID FIRE

1. I have a leathery, rough skin texture. How to make it smooth?

Use a chemical exfoliant. You may also opt for procedures like chemical peels, microdermabrasion, micro-needling and skin boosters. Refer to the chapter on exfoliation and active ingredients for the same.

2. I have ugly scars on my face which look like craters. These occurred when my acne healed and I was very depressed and had lost my self-confidence in my twenties and thirties due to these scars. Now I have learnt to live with them and am fifty but I see my son getting acne like me. What can be done to prevent him from developing scars like mine?

Please make sure he doesn't pick at them. Most importantly, start medication and treatment for active acne as soon as you see acne. Early intervention is the only way to prevent scars.

3. I have been seeing four tiny black spots on my hands since a few months. The doctors said they are harmless moles. Can we get moles at the age of thirty-five?

Yes, moles can occur at any age and your doctor is right.

4. I see pink and violet streaks on my thighs and shoulders. They look like stretch marks, but I know that stretch marks are usually white in colour. What could these be?

Newly formed stretch marks are pink or violet or reddish in colour. They gradually turn white as the scarring increases.

5. What is the quickest way to get a smooth skin texture?

Unfortunately, none. Please consult with a dermatologist to works towards smooth and radiant skin. It's possible but it takes a few months.

17

Skin Tone

'Surely god was biased when he made you in shades of dark brown. Remember eumelanin which is responsible for dark colour protects you from UV radiation and prevents skin cancer. Embrace your skin colour.'

—Dr Jaishree Sharad

The colour of your skin is most often referred to as skin tone and is determined by the amount of and type of pigment melanin present in your skin. This hugely depends on your genetic makeup, ethnicity and ancestral origin. Melanin is produced by cells called melanocytes present in the skin. There are two types of melanin which determine the colour of your skin and hair, namely eumelanin and phaeomelanin. When there is more eumelanin and less phaeomelanin, the colour of the skin is dark. When there is more phaeomelanin and less eumelanin, the skin is lighter in colour. Eumelanin, which is responsible for dark colour, protects us from UV radiation-induced molecular damage. Eumelanin also prevents the skin from developing skin cancer and deep wrinkles. Phaeomelanin, present in higher concentration in fair skin actually becomes a free radical and aggravates the damage caused by light.

1. What is hyperpigmentation?

When the skin colour darkens as compared to the natural skin tone, it is called hyperpigmentation. Hyperpigmentation is a benign and harmless condition, and is quite common. It can be seen in patches or over a large area of the skin or entire body.

2. Are there any skin-lightening agents for hyperpigmentation?

Hydroquinone is a commonly used skin-lightening agent, which should be used under the strict supervision of a dermatologist. Hydroxy acids are also used, which work by exfoliation of the skin cells and sloughing off the build-up, thus reducing hyperpigmentation. Vitamins such as vitamin A and its derivatives such as retinoids cause exfoliation and prevent melanin pigment formation. Vitamin B3, also known as niacinamide, and vitamin C are popular ingredients in skin-lightening products as they inhibit pigment formation. Vitamins C and E are powerful antioxidants, which fight free radicals and help in reducing pigmentation. Steroids available over the counter as skin-lightening creams are often used by people without prescription and can lead to side effects such as

242 The Skincare Answer Book

thinning of skin, pimples, poor wound healing, broken capillaries and increased risk of infection. Avoid creams containing fluticasone, flucinolone, betamethasone, clobetasol, hydrocortisone and mometasone.

3. What is the role of botanicals in the treatment of hyperpigmentation?

Botanical products are becoming more popular as skin-lightening agents as they have minimal side effects and a high safety profile. Most of them are antioxidant skin lighteners. Products such as kojic acid, alpha arbutin, liquorice (glabridin), soy, pycnogenol, coffee berry, tomato (lycopene), grape seed extract, orchid extract, aloe vera extract, marine algae extract, cinnamic acid, flavonoids, green tea extract, aloesin, mulberry extract and emblica are some of the botanicals used in the treatment of hyperpigmentation.

4. What are chemical peels? What are fruit peels? Can they be done to reduce hyperpigmentation?

Chemical peeling is a procedure that involves the application of a solution to the skin in a controlled manner, producing controlled tissue damage. The solution may be an acid, a fruit extract, a botanical extract or even a milk extract. The type of peel is decided by the doctor depending on the skin and the cause of pigmentation. All fruit peels are chemical peels because they are extracts of a fruit with added preservatives and chemicals.

Chemical peels can be used to reduce pigmentation. Some of the peels that help reduce pigmentation are AHA peels such as glycolic acid, which is derived from sugarcane or lactic acid, which is derived from fermented milk, yoghurt and tomatoes or Mandelic acid derived from bitter almonds, peaches and apricots. Lactic acid maintains the skin's pH level and also moisturizes the skin. Other peels including those using arginine, which is derived from brown sugar; kojic acid, which is derived from a few species of the fungus Aspergillus, TCA, which is derived from trichloroacetic acid; and tretinoin, which is derived from retinoic acid, a vitamin A derivative, also help reduce hyperpigmentation.

5. What are the side effects of peels?

Chemical peeling has side effects if the candidate, the peel and the method of application are not right. Also, if the aftercare is not proper, there is increased risk of redness, swelling, flaking and increased hyperpigmentation, which may last up to a week. Hence always get peels done by a professional.

6. Can Laser help reduce hyperpigmentation?

Yes, certain types of hyperpigmentation are treated with Q-switched Nd:YAG Laser and Pico Laser. Six to eight sessions at six-weekly intervals are normally recommended. But Laser should be used with caution. Improper use may cause darkening of the skin. Be sure to consult a dermatologist and let them diagnose your condition and conduct the procedure for the same.

7. Does vitamin C reduce hyperpigmentation?

Yes, vitamin C helps reduce hyperpigmentation as it is a potent antioxidant. It fights free radicals and reduces the formation of melanin.

8. Are there any dietary guidelines that can help reduce pigmentation?

A diet rich in antioxidants, which can combat the harmful effects of UV rays, can help. Brightly coloured fruits and vegetables, green tea, soy, and vitamins A, C and E are rich in antioxidants so including them in your diet will be beneficial.

9. What are the dos and don'ts of hyperpigmentation?

Use a sunscreen with SPF50 indoors as well as outdoors, and reapply every two to three hours. Avoid constantly wiping your skin. It is better to avoid using hair colour with paraphenylenediamine (PPD), and you can also refrain from using perfumes and foundations to see if your condition improves. Get your insulin resistance, sugar and hormone levels tested. It is best to consult a dermatologist for proper guidance. The eight S's that can increase hyperpigmentation are sunlight, smoking, stress, sugar, swimming outdoors in daylight, steam and sauna, scent and scrubs. So it is best to avoid them if you suffer from hyperpigmentation.

10. I have heard about glutathione injections and that they make the skin fair. How safe are they and how often can I take them? Will glutathione tablets also make me fair?

Glutathione is a potent antioxidant that is given for liver detoxification to patients with alcoholic liver disease, liver cirrhosis and fatty liver. The usual dose is 600 to 1200 mg. It can reduce melanin to a certain extent, but skin whitening is more of a side effect of glutathione.

So, not everybody becomes fairer with the use of glutathione. Second, in those people who experience skin lightening, the effect may wear off once they stop taking glutathione. Tablets or capsules of 500 to 1000 mg are also available and can be taken safely for about three months as potent antioxidants and not skin-lightening agents.

DARK CIRCLES

1. What are the causes of dark circles?

There are various causes of dark circles. One of the most common reasons is lack of sleep. It creates sunken eyes, which forms a shadow around the eyes, resulting in the formation of dark circles. Post-inflammatory hyperpigmentation (PIH) caused by frequent rubbing of the eyes is another factor responsible for dark circles. This may be due to habit, dry skin or eczema. The extension of pigmentary demarcation lines could also lead to the formation of dark circles. Genetics could also be a factor and may even be evident from childhood itself. Health conditions such as low haemoglobin, diabetes or insulin resistance, superficial blood vessels in the skin and allergies to cosmetics, hair colour, fragrance, pollution, dust, etc. could also cause dark circles. Other factors such as smoking, stress and excessive exposure to sun can also lead to the formation of dark circles.

2. How does one treat dark circles?

The skin under the eyes is very thin and needs to be moisturized regularly. You must also apply a sunscreen under your eyes during the day and wear sunglasses that are UV protective. Response to treatments for dark circles is slow and can take up to one to two years. It also requires maintenance with lifestyle changes and use of topical creams or serums. Using creams helps prevent the dark circles from getting worse. Creams containing vitamin C, vitamin K, liquorice, arbutin, kojic acid, soy and other skin-lightening botanicals can be used if you have dark circles. You will have to use the cream for at least six months before you can expect to see results. Chemical peeling using peeling agents such as glycolic acid, lactic acid, arginine, etc., strictly done at a skin clinic, may also help. However, multiple sessions will be needed to see results. Lasers such as Q-switched Nd:YAG and Pico wave are also used to treat the pigmentary and vascular components of dark circles. Usually, six to ten sessions are needed with the interval between two sessions being six to eight weeks. A combination of treatments or stepwise treatments planned by your dermatologist will benefit you more.

Make sure you sleep for six to eight hours every night and avoid frequent late nights. Quit smoking and meditate or do pranayam to help in coping with stress. Avoid rubbing your eyes often. Get eye allergies treated if you have any since eye allergies may result in itching which will indirectly lead to dark circles due to constant friction. If you are allergic to dust, smoke, etc., wear a mask when you are outdoors. Get treated if you suffer from hay fever, asthma and nasal congestion. If you have low haemoglobin, take iron supplements. Never forget to moisturize the skin under the eyes, especially if you have eczema or atopic dermatitis.

Avoid using cosmetics that are over six months old and avoid wearing kajal, mascara, eyeliner and eyeshadow if you are allergic to them. If at all you do wear them, be gentle while cleansing and removing them.

3. I am only nineteen years old, and I have very bad dark circles in spite of sleeping for ten hours every night. How can I get rid of my dark circles?

Dark circles can occur at any age, and they are not always related to lack of sleep, although that is the most common cause. You need to first identify the cause and treat it. Sometimes dark circles are genetic and may be evident from childhood itself.

4. My eyes look hollow and tired, and it appears as if I haven't slept for ages even though I sleep well. I have dark circles too. What is the best treatment for me?

The bone around the eyes known as the orbital rim comprises the frontal and the maxillary bone. These bones may be genetically concave or there may be bone degeneration with age. This, along with less fat, leads to sunken eyes or hollows under the eyes. Medically, this is called the tear trough deformity. When light falls under the eye it casts a shadow, which looks like dark circles. When you stretch the skin you will notice that there are actually no dark circles, and it is only a shadow that makes the under-eye area look dull, tired and haggard. The best treatment option for hollow under-eyes is hyaluronic acid filler injections. Hyaluronic acid is a safe, US Food and Drug Administration (FDA)-approved filler and is most forgiving since it can be dissolved with a hyaluronidase injection should you not like the effect of the filler. The effect lasts for one to two years and can be repeated safely. Hyaluronic acid is also biostimulatory, i.e., it stimulates skin cells called fibroblasts to produce newer collagen. So with time, the filler begins to last longer and the need to refill every year reduces. The other option is to inject autologous micro fat grafts. The fat is taken from one's abdomen or thigh, centrifuged and the micro fat graft collected is injected in the under-eye area. This procedure is either performed by a qualified dermatosurgeon, cosmetic surgeon or oculoplastic surgeon.

5. At what age can I start doing under-eye fillers?

If you have a genetic deformity, you can even start at the age of twenty-two. The US FDA has approved the use of under-eye fillers for anyone above the age of eighteen. We must understand that the sooner we start, the better it is to prevent worsening of the condition.

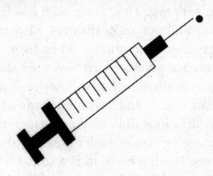

6. Is there a specific type of filler that can be injected under the eye?

One must opt for very light or low G prime hyaluronic acid fillers under the eye. Always correct the under-eye hollow since hyaluronic acid absorbs water and swells up.

7. How can I prevent fine lines and sagging skin under my eyes?

Moisturize the skin twice a day and always apply a sunscreen. Use a vitamin C serum under your moisturizer and sunscreen during the day and a serum containing retinol, AHA or peptides under the eye at bedtime. You may also opt for treatments such as microneedling with platelet-rich plasma or skin booster injections (both have been described in chapter on skin aging).

8. Are there any home remedies for dark circles?

None of the home remedies really help in getting rid of dark circles completely, but they may temporarily make the dark circles look less prominent. Application of cucumber slices over the eyes and relaxing for about ten to twenty minutes can help. You may also do this with refrigerated tea bags as caffeine is known to have skin-lightening effects. You may try applying a few drops of cold milk at bedtime. Milk contains lactic acid, which has both moisturizing as well as skin-lightening properties. Do not try applying lemon juice or tomato slices as these are acidic and may sometimes irritate the thin skin around the eyes and cause post-inflammatory hyperpigmentation.

9. My eyelids are very dark. What can be done to lighten them?

You can follow the same regimen that applies for the under-eye area. Moisturize, apply sunscreen, vitamin C serum and skin-lightening creams with liquorice or arbutin, etc. Microneedling with Dermapen and a needle depth of 0.2 mm may be done on the upper eyelid. However, chemical peels and Lasers are not done on the upper eyelid skin.

10. I have puffy eyes, and it runs in my family. How can I reduce the puffiness?

Puffy eyes can either be physiological, that is due to lifestyle or could be the result of a fat prolapse, which is either genetic or due to age. In cases of mild fat herniation, we may inject very light hyaluronic acid fillers under the eyes in very small quantities to camouflage the puffiness. In cases of severe fat prolapse, under-eye blepharoplasty is the only way out. Physiological puffy

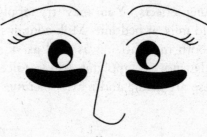

Puffy eyes

eyes can occur due to fluid retention under the eyes due to poor lymphatic drainage, consuming alcohol or a salty diet or even smoking. Lifestyle changes must be made to reduce puffy eyes, especially when one wakes up in the morning.

There are various ways to reduce puffy eyes. One of them is to reduce your salt intake. Salt is never good in high amounts, and if you love eating salty foods but are having consistent problems with bags under the eyes, chances are your salt intake is to blame. Eating too much salt can make your body retain more water. It can also depress the blood circulation in your body, causing puffiness around the eyes. Similarly, it is best to avoid gluten, dairy, sugar and alcohol. Allergies or intolerance to any of these can result in puffy eyes in the morning. Another big thing you can do to prevent bags from forming is to increase the amount of vitamin K you're getting. Leafy greens such as kale and Swiss chard contain high amounts of vitamin K and can greatly help in preventing bags. Eating a small salad every day full of greens is an easy way to make sure you're getting enough of this vitamin. Also, look for under-eye creams that contain vitamin K so that the vitamin will absorb directly into the problematic area. Using your fingers, a guasha or a jade roller to massage the face and drain the lymphatic fluid also reduces puffiness. Avoiding allergens whenever you can will also help prevent puffy eyes. You may not have allergies per say, but allergens can also be the cause of puffy eyes. Sleeping with your head raised helps prevent puffiness too. It may not be the most comfortable position for many people, but sleeping on your back with your head raised is a great way to prevent puffy eyes as you're preventing blood from pooling around the eyes. Smoking is another cause of bags under the eyes. The nicotine in cigarettes can limit the body's ability to circulate blood, which can have a direct effect on the circulation around your eyes. Hence it's best to avoid smoking.

DARK LIPS

1. What are the causes of dark lips?

The outer covering of the lips, known as the lip mucosa, does not contain stratified squamous cell epithelium and a protective barrier layer like the skin. Hence it is more prone to damage and injury, leading to discoloration. Injury to the lips or allergies can cause inflammation of the lip mucosa, which results in hyperpigmentation or darkening of the lips. Some of the common causes are allergy to the ingredients in lipsticks, lip balms, lip glosses and lip plumpers, allergy to perfumes, nail varnish, toothpaste, mouth fresheners, silver-coated condiments, and allergy to certain drugs such as amiodarone, daunorubicin, gold, methotrexate, psoralens and 5-flurouracil. Allergies to some drugs such as painkillers and antibiotics can result in Fixed drug eruptions which are seen as violaceous dark spots on lips. Cold climates and prolonged exposure to air conditioning, frequent lip licking, lip biting, smoking, vaping, using Juul, chewing tobacco, lip eczema or skin disorders such as lichen planus, and frequent lip scrubbing or exfoliation can also cause dark lips.

2. Can lipsticks cause dark lips?

If you have dark lips, you must avoid lip plumpers, long-lasting lipsticks, lipsticks of poor quality and very dark colours such as dark browns, dark reds or dark maroons. People who suffer from lip eczema or dark lips could be allergic to the ingredients present in lipsticks, lip glosses or lip plumpers. Some of the common ingredients that can cause allergies are emollients such as ricinoleic acid, castor oil, sesame oil, ozonated olive oil, coconut oil, colophony, shellac and preservatives like propyl gallate. Sometimes the elements used for fragrance and flavour such as Balsam of Peru, citral, geraniol, vanilla, fragrance mix, cinnamaldehyde and peppermint oil can also cause allergies. The elements used for colour such as D&C Yellow #11; D&C Red #7, #17, #21 (eosin) and #36; Lithol Rubine BCA; and quinazoline yellow, as well as the nickel from the metal casing may also be responsible for allergies. So, your lip products should be devoid of these ingredients.

3. I don't smoke, so why are my lips dark? How can I lighten dark lips?

Smoking is not the only cause of dark lips. There are many other reasons as listed above. You need to identify the cause and eliminate it.

You can follow some of these tips to help lighten your lips. Avoid pursing or licking your lips. Carry a lip cream with you and keep applying it every two hours if you have dry, chapped lips. Drink 2–3 litres of water to avoid dehydration. You can also keep lips hydrated by applying ghee, petroleum jelly or fragrance-free lip balms. Avoid lip cosmetics as far as possible and if you have to use them, do not use lip cosmetics that are over six months old. Avoid using dark shades of lipstick and unknown brands and avoid fragrance-based lip glosses and lip plumpers. Use good old white-coloured toothpastes or check with your dermatologist. Avoid all mints and sweets with silver coating. Do not use perfume and nail varnishes if you have sensitive skin or a known allergy to them. You can use lip-lightening creams containing kojic acid, liquorice extract, niacinamide, arbutin, mulberry, vitamin C or vitamin E. Lactic or glycolic acid peels also help to lighten lip colour. Persistent dark colour may be treated with Q-switched Nd:YAG Laser or a Pico Laser. Do not try creams or treatments without consulting a dermatologist.

4. Can you suggest some home remedies for dark lips?

Always keep your lips hydrated. You can apply ghee on your lips. A paste of sugar, turmeric and yoghurt applied for about ten minutes then washed off may help. Avoid scrubbing with lemon, sugar, etc. as vigorous exfoliation can damage the lip mucosa.

5. What creams can I use for dark lips?

Creams containing kojic acid, arbutin, mulberry extract, azelaic acid, aloesin, liquorice, soy, green tea, lignin peroxidase, niacinamide, ellagic acid, turmeric, ascorbic

Scheman A, Jacob S, Zirwas M, et al. Contact allergy: alternatives for the 2007 North American contact dermatitis group (NACDG) Standard Screening Tray. Dis Mon. 2008;54(1-2):7–156

Lalko J, Api AM. Investigation of the dermal sensitization potential of various essential oils in the local lymph node assay. Food Chem Toxicol. 2006;44(5):739–746. Epub 2005 Dec 1.

Frosch PJ, Johansen JD, Menné T, et al. Further important sensitizers in patients sensitive to fragrances. Contact Dermatitis. 2002;47(5): 279–287.

acid, coffee berry, vitamin C and vitamin E help in lightening lips.

6. Can Laser lighten dark lips permanently?

Yes, eight to ten sessions of Q-switched Nd:YAG Laser or fewer sessions of Pico Laser can reduce hyperpigmentation. The interval between two sessions should be four to eight weeks.

7. Is lip blushing a good option for dark lips?

It is difficult to match the lip shade when using permanent lip colour if your lips are dark.

8. What is lip blushing and how safe is it?

Lip blushing is a form of semi-permanent make-up. It is done by tattooing the lips with semi-permanent colour to improve the colour, shape and definition of the lips. A motorized device with a tiny sterile needle is used to deposit pigment into the lips, which builds layers of colour. It is similar to microblading of eyebrows. Lip blushing can last several years, but touch-ups are needed every six to eight months. Smoking, sun exposure, lip allergies, exfoliation, etc. can speed up the fading process. Sometimes people develop allergies to the pigment deposited in the lips, and sometimes they may develop infections if the device and needles are not sterile. One needs to make sure that the needle is exclusively used for them and disposed to prevent infections like HIV, herpes labialis and hepatitis B.

DARK ELBOWS, KNEES AND ANKLES

1. Why are my elbows, ankles and knees dark?

Darkening of elbows, ankles and knees is a common phenomenon especially among people with darker skin tone. One of the most common causes is constant friction. The frequent rubbing of elbows and knees against something makes the skin thicker and darker in colour than the surrounding area. If you are on your knees a lot or often sit with your legs folded, rest your elbows on the table or use a loofah, pumice stone or scrub every day on these areas, there will be darkening of skin due to friction. Build-up of dead skin cells or dirt can also make your knees, ankles and elbows darker. Excessive exposure to sunlight can stimulate over-production of melanin, causing pigmentation. Sometimes a hormonal imbalance such as in cases of diabetes, polycystic ovarian syndrome, hypothyroidism, etc. can also result in dark elbows, ankles and knees. Certain skin disorders like atopic dermatitis cause a lot of dryness, also resulting in darkening of elbows, ankles and knees.

2. How can one lighten one's elbows, knees and ankles?

A little darkening of these areas is normal. Avoid constant friction and tight clothing. Make sure you use a good moisturizer followed by a sunscreen with SPF30. Use a moisturizer with oils, waxes, lanolin, dimethicone and ceramides and moisturize the elbows, knees and ankles at least two to three times per day. Gentle exfoliation once a week with a soft cloth will remove dead skin accumulation. Do not exfoliate with loofahs or pumice stones. Alternatively, you can use a gentle chemical exfoliator that contains AHA or BHA every other night. These are usually well tolerated by most people. Use pigment-lightening creams with ingredients such as kojic acid, vitamin C, retinoids, 2 per cent hydroquinone, azelaic acid, glycolic acid or salicylic acid. However, it is best to consult a dermatologist before you use these. Avoid using bleaching creams or products containing mercury. Some of them, such as retinol and salicylic acid, are unsafe during pregnancy. Give it at least three to four months to see an improvement. If the dark colour persists, you could visit a dermatologist for skin-lightening peels. You can opt for salicylic, retinol, phenol and TCA peels. About six to eight sessions at three-week intervals will reduce the discolouration.

3. Are there any home remedies for dark knees, elbows and ankles?

You can try the following do-it-yourself tricks. Take two teaspoons of chickpea flour and make a paste. Add a pinch of turmeric and a tablespoon of yoghurt. Apply this mixture to the elbows, knees, knuckles and ankles. Leave this on for thirty minutes and then wash thoroughly. Immediately dab a moisturizer on slightly damp skin to lock in the moisture. Do this every alternate day for a couple of weeks to reduce the dark colour. Chickpea flour is a good cleanser, moisturizer and skin lightener and turmeric is an antiseptic, which helps reduce the discolouration. You can also take a teaspoon of sugar, add crushed oats and mashed papaya and leave the mixture on the elbows, ankles and knees for about ten minutes and then rinse it off. Follow it with a good moisturizer.

4. How do I prevent my knees, elbows and ankles from getting dark?

You should avoid putting pressure on the knees, ankles and elbows for extended periods of time. Make a conscious effort to avoid sitting cross-legged. Make sure you do not wear clothes that are tight around the elbows, ankles and knees. Avoid resting your elbows on the table or chair for too long. Always moisturize your elbows, knees and ankles thoroughly at least twice a day followed by a sunscreen with SPF30. Gentle exfoliation once a week with a soft cloth helps remove dead skin accumulation. However, excessive exfoliation can be counter-productive and worsen the skin darkening. Avoid harsh scrubs, pumice stone and loofahs. Avoid using bleaching creams. Lack of vitamins A and E can adversely affect your skin and cause dark patches, so you should take vitamin A and vitamin E in your diet. You must include vegetables like carrots, sweet potatoes, pumpkin, etc. in your diet for vitamin A, and nuts like almonds hazelnuts, peanuts and sunflower seeds and greens like spinach for vitamin E.

DARK KNUCKLES

1. Why are my knuckles dark?

Dark knuckles can occur due to skin conditions such as acanthosis nigricans, which causes thick, dark, velvety skin. Pre-diabetic people who are at the risk of acanthosis nigricans can also develop dark knuckles. People with hormonal conditions like polycystic ovarian syndrome and those who have a vitamin B12 deficiency can also have dark knuckles. Rare skin diseases like dermatomyositis, which causes muscle weakness, can lead to the formation of bluish-purple rashes on the knuckles, elbows, heels and toes. Underlying cancer can also cause dark knuckles. Drug reaction due to NSAIDs or antibiotics, and an allergy to detergents or chemicals that cause contact dermatitis can lead to pigmentation of the knuckles. Other factors such as constant friction due to scrubbing and sports such as boxing can also cause dark knuckles.

2. How can I get rid of dark knuckles?

The underlying cause should be identified and treated. Use a vitamin C serum, followed by a thick moisturizer and sunscreen every morning. At night, apply depigmenting creams containing azelaic acid, glycolic acid, arbutin and retinoids. Consult a dermatologist who can prescribe the right cream for you depending on the type of hyperpigmentation. In-clinic chemical peels using glycolic acid or TCA can help. Q-switched Nd:YAG Laser is another in-clinic treatment option.

3. Are there any home remedies for dark knuckles?

Curd is a moisturizer and skin lightener, so you can apply curd, or you can add mashed papaya to it and apply the mixture on dark knuckles, leave it on for ten minutes and then wash it off. You can do this daily for a few weeks. Milk and milk cream contain lactic acid, which can be used to lighten dark knuckles. Take a teaspoon of milk and add two teaspoons of honey. Make a paste and apply it over dark knuckles. Let it dry and then wash it off. You can also use milk cream and add a pinch of turmeric powder to it, make a paste and apply it over your knuckles. Leave it on for ten to fifteen minutes, then wash it off. Aloe vera gel obtained from the central core of the leaf can be applied on dark knuckles. Almond oil and sandalwood oil have bleaching effects and can thus help lighten dark knuckles.

4. How do I prevent my knuckles from getting dark?

Keep your knuckles soft and moisturized. Every time you wash your hands you should apply a moisturizer.

DARK UNDERARMS

1. Why are my armpits so dark?

Underarms or armpits, also known as axilla in medical terminology, can be dark due to various reasons:

- Allergies to deodorants and perfumes: Fragrances, paraben, alcohol, etc. are known to cause allergies and inflammation, resulting in the darkening of underarm skin.
- Fungal, yeast or bacterial infections: Candida and Corynebacterium minutissimum are some common infections that occur in the folds of the skin such as the underarms, groin and elbow folds. Sweat from sweat glands and apocrine glands in the body harbour these microorganisms and thus excessive sweating can cause dark armpits.

- Friction due to shaving or waxing: Repeated friction due to shaving or waxing can result in irritation of the skin. This causes melanocytes (pigment cells) in the skin to multiply at an unusually rapid rate, resulting in darkening of the skin.
- Post-inflammatory hyperpigmentation: When infections, allergies or skin conditions such as lichen planus and hidradenitis suppurativa subside, there is excess production of melanin by the melanocytes, resulting in hyperpigmentation.
- Friction: Tight-fitting clothes, especially those made with synthetic fabrics, can cause excessive friction, resulting in dark underarms. Frequent exfoliation can also result in friction-induced darkening of skin.
- Hormonal issues: Insulin resistance, PCOS, hypothyroidism, diabetes, hyperprolactinemia or Addison's disease may result in darkening of the skin, especially at the body folds.
- Obesity: Repeated rubbing of skin in body folds can cause darkening. Moreover, in most people who are obese, high levels of the hormone insulin in the blood can result in a condition called acanthosis nigricans and thus darkening.
- Acanthosis nigricans: In people who have insulin resistance, diabetes or PCOS, the skin in the body folds becomes thick, velvety and dark. This condition is known as acanthosis nigricans, commonly seen in the neck, underarms, elbow creases and under the breasts.
- Smoking: This is a common cause of hyperpigmentation. The pigment melanin in the skin increases due to smoking and results in darkening.

2. Can obesity cause dark underarms?

Yes, those who are overweight can develop dark underarms either due to friction or they may be suffering from an underlying hormonal condition such as insulin resistance, hypothyroidism or PCOS.

3. How can one lighten dark underarms?

Identify the cause and eliminate it or get it treated. If you have infections or allergies, consult a dermatologist and get them treated. If you have any hormonal issues, get them checked and treated. If your BMI is more than 25, you should work towards losing weight. Instead of deodorants, use antifungal powder. If you do use perfumes, avoid spraying them directly on your skin and instead spray them on your clothes. Wear loose-fitting cotton to deal with sweating. If you sweat excessively, you may opt for botulinum toxin injections available as Botox, Xeomin or Dysport. Another option for excessive sweating is treatment with a device called miraDry, which uses microwave technology to reduce sweating. Go for Laser hair removal instead of shaving or waxing. Using salicylic acid or AHA peels. Q-switched Nd:YAG Lasers can also help. Apply pigment-lightening creams only on the advice of your dermatologist.

4. Will underarm darkening go away if I stop shaving?

If the darkening is due to shaving, it is better to stop shaving and opt for Laser hair removal. This will prevent further darkening. However, you will need to get the darkening treated by a dermatologist.

5. Does deodorant cause dark armpits?

A study showed that 60 to 70 per cent of individuals were detected with fragrance allergy. The common fragrances that result in darkening of skin are Balsam of Peru, Lyral, tea tree oil, arnica montana, lichen acid mix, Lavender Absolute, essential oils like geraniol, eugenol, citral, ylang-ylang oil and lemongrass. Propylene glycol, a solvent with moisturizing, antiseptic and preservative properties, was the second most commonly present allergen and was present in 47 per cent of the deodorants contained in the Walgreens database.

6. What should I use to combat sweating or odour if deodorants are causing dark underarms?

Deodorants can cause dark underarms, so instead use an antifungal powder just after your bath on absolutely dry skin as maintaining good hygiene is extremely important. Also, make sure you change clothes every day. Sweat, dirt and sebum, which seep into your clothes when you wear them, remain in the clothes and result in a foul odour. You can also use antiperspirants. Antiperspirant solution containing aluminium chloride hexahydrate is often used. However, sometimes antiperspirants can lead to irritation and can even clog pores. Excessive sweating can be treated with diluted doses of botulinum toxin injected into the underarms. The other option for excessive sweating is treatment with a device called miraDry, which is based on radio frequency microwave technology.

7. How can I lighten my underarms naturally?

Try using a mix of yoghurt and turmeric for a couple of weeks. If it helps, you are lucky. If it doesn't, you need to see a dermatologist. Do not scrub your underarms with loofahs, beads, fruit extracts, etc. Scrubbing will only increase the pigmentation.

8. Can one reverse underarm darkening?

With treatment by using skin-lightening creams, chemical peels and Q-switched Nd:YAG Laser dark underarms will appear lighter.

9. Can dark underarms be due to hormonal conditions?

Yes, hormonal conditions such as polycystic ovarian disease and hypothyroidism can cause underarm darkening. Insulin resistance eventually leads to diabetes and increases the likelihood of acanthosis nigricans thus leading to dark underarms.

DARK FOREHEAD

1. What are the causes of a hyperpigmented forehead or forehead darkening?

The common causes of darkening of the forehead are:

- Sun exposure: This is the most common cause. The forehead is the area most prone to sun exposure. Excessive sun exposure causes more melanin production thus resulting in hyperpigmentation.
- Irritant contact dermatitis due to use of balms for headaches or colds: Balms that claim to relieve

headaches are counter-irritants. They contain menthol, camphor, peppermint, cajaput oil and clove oil, which can irritate the skin and cause hyperpigmentation. Stop using balms if you have pigmentation or even the slightest history of pigmentation.

- Friction: Constant friction due to wiping of sweat, using thick Turkish napkins, etc. can result in hyperpigmentation.
- Allergy to hair colours: Hair colours may look good on your hair but if your skin is allergic to them, they are not worth it. Hair colours have an ingredient called Paraphenylenediamine (PPD), which is the most common allergen. People may develop blisters on their scalp, an itchy scalp or pigmentation along the hairline, which gradually spreads to the rest of the face.
- Allergy to fragrances: Perfumes can cause pigmentation or increase existing pigmentation. Fragrance in a jar, bottle, bar or powder in the form of cosmetics, perfumes, soaps and talcum powder can cause hyperpigmentation.
- Drug-induced pigmentation: Pigmentation resulting after the use of unknown drugs and powders given by sadhus is seen due to the presence of heavy metals (lead, mercury, silver, gold and bismuth). Antimalarials, anti-cancer drugs, minocycline, psoralens as well as many antidepressant and anti-anxiety drugs can also cause hyperpigmentation.
- Smoking and stress: Smoking and stress increase the free radicals in your skin, leading to an increase in hyperpigmentation.

- Nutritional deficiency: Deficiency of vitamins B12 and B3 (niacin) can cause darkening of skin.
- Other causes could be genetic, health conditions such as acanthosis nigricans due to insulin resistance, diabetes and thyroid disorder. Overly aggressive skincare treatments can also cause hyperpigmentation.

2. What are the home remedies for a hyperpigmented forehead?

You can try a yoghurt and turmeric mask. Two teaspoons of yoghurt mixed with a pinch of turmeric can be applied on the forehead for thirty minutes and then washed off. You can do this once every couple of weeks. Yoghurt contains lactic acid, which is a natural skin bleach and moisturizer. Turmeric is an antibacterial and skin lightener with powerful antioxidants. (Those who are allergic to turmeric should not use this mask.) Another option is a potato and tomato mask. Extract the juice from a crushed potato and add it to a mashed tomato. Apply this mixture over blemishes and dark patches. Leave it on for twenty minutes and then wash it off. Potatoes contain a high amount of catecholase, a potent skin-lightening substance. Tomatoes are rich in lycopene and vitamin C, both powerful antioxidants. The mixture works on hyperpigmentation and helps reduce dark patches.

3. How can one prevent hyperpigmentation on the forehead?

There could be various causes for hyperpigmentation. Fragrance can be a cause. Any fragrance in a jar, bottle, bar or powder can cause hyperpigmentation. Hence if you use perfume, for instance, spray it on your clothes and then wear them after ten minutes. Similarly, if you wear make-up, opt for mineral powder instead of foundation. Avoid using balms on your forehead often. Use them only if your headache or cold worsens. Refrain from using hair colour with PPD. You can opt for an organic hair colour or vegetable dye instead. Henna can also be used, but conditioning is required to tackle dryness of hair post henna application. Avoid the use of nylon brushes or loofahs to scrub the dirt off your body and the use of thick Turkish napkins. Instead, use soft napkins to wipe sweat as this helps avoid friction and thus reduces pigmentation. Exposure to intense heat could also lead to hyperpigmentation. So avoid heat in the kitchen from the stove, steam and sauna rooms or relaxing hot yoga sessions as they can actually increase pigmentation. Stress and smoking can increase free radical production and thus lead to pigmentation. Hence think before you smoke and learn or pursue a hobby you enjoy to destress. Practising yoga and meditation can also help. Apart from these, do test your insulin levels to determine the cause of hyperpigmentation.

DARK ARMS, LEGS AND BACK

1. What are the causes of dark arms, legs and back?

There could be various causes. One of the most common is excessive sun exposure over a period of time. This causes melanin production, resulting in hyperpigmentation. Another reason could be macular amyloidosis. It is seen as dark, mottled, pigmented spots on the arms, forearms and upper back. These patches occur due to the accumulation of abnormal proteins, known as amyloids, in the skin. Sometimes this condition is genetic. But often, the abnormal protein deposition leading to pigmentation is induced by prolonged use of nylon scrubs, nylon brushes, loofahs, pumice stone, synthetic scrubs, thick towels, plant sticks and leaves. Nutritional deficiency such as deficiency of vitamins B12 and B3 (niacin) can also cause darkening of skin on the body. Pigmentation can also be drug-induced. Consuming unknown drugs and powders in the name of Ayurveda that may not be pure can result in pigmentation due to the presence of heavy metals (lead, mercury, silver, gold and bismuth). Antimalarials, anti-cancer drugs, minocycline, psoralens, antidepressant and antianxiety drugs may cause hyperpigmentation. Keratosis pilaris can also cause pigmentation. It is caused by keratin accumulation in the hair follicles and seen as tiny dark dots on the arms, sometimes leaving a rough texture. They may sometimes be seen on the legs too. Allergic contact dermatitis, eczemas and skin conditions like lichen planus pigmentosus can also lead to post-inflammatory hyperpigmentation. Allergy to fragrance (fragrance in incense sticks, room diffusers, perfumes, deodorants, skincare products, etc.) can also cause pigmentation or increase existing pigmentation. Some autoimmune conditions such as hypothyroidism, and diabetes too can result in the darkening of skin.

2. How does one treat hyperpigmentation on the arms and back?

The most important precaution is to always apply sunscreen with SPF50 on all exposed parts of the body and wear full-sleeved clothes from sunrise to sunset. Moisturize twice a day and avoid the use of nylon loofahs, brushes, pumice stones, etc. for scrubbing as this can also increase hyperpigmentation. Check your thyroid hormones, insulin and blood sugar levels and get treated in case of abnormal hormone levels. Skin-lightening creams, topical corticosteroids, calcineurin inhibitors such as tacrolimus and pimecrolimus may also be used as prescribed by the dermatologist.

3. Which peels can be done to reduce the darkening on the arms, legs and back?

TCA, glycolic acid, salicylic acid, lactic acid and retinol peels can be done to reduce pigmentation in dark patches on the arms, legs and back.

4. What home remedies can one try to lighten the arms, legs and back?

Usually home remedies do not work unless it is a tan. You can apply yoghurt with honey and keep it on for ten to fifteen minutes before washing it off. This can be done once every couple of weeks. Yoghurt contains lactic acid, which is a natural skin bleacher and moisturizer, while honey is a soothing agent preventing inflammation. Fresh aloe vera gel can also be applied for ten to fifteen minutes and rinsed off. Aloe vera contains aloin, which is a natural depigmenting agent. It is anti-inflammatory and provides hydration.

5. How long does it take to clear up hyperpigmentation? Does application of skin-lightening agents reduce the time taken?

If the dark spots are superficial, in the epidermis, they may fade over three months. If there is uniform dark pigmentation, it may take eight months to one year for it to fade away even with treatment. Some conditions such as macular amyloidosis or keratosis pilaris can only be controlled and the pigmentation can only be lightened. It may not disappear completely. Skin-lightening agents such as retinols, AHAs and BHAs will hasten the process, whereas vitamins C and E prevent melanin formation and prevent existing pigment from getting darker.

DARK FEET

1. My feet, especially my toes, have become very dark. What should I do?

Sun exposure, post-inflammatory hyperpigmentation (PIH), allergy to shoes (leather, plastic, rubber), eczema, dry skin, hemosiderin staining and constant use of loofah scrubs can cause dark feet.

Use a broad-spectrum sunscreen daily. Wear cotton socks to avoid direct contact with your shoes in case you are allergic to leather or rubber. Wear well-fitted shoes that do not cause any friction. Avoid scrubbing your feet. Moisturize your feet well. Use skin-lightening creams as prescribed by your dermatologist.

2. I am twenty-eight years old and have dark pigmentation around the corners of my nose and on my chin crease below my lower lip. Sometimes it flakes and other times there is a whitish discharge if I squeeze the skin.

You seem to be suffering from a condition called seborrhoeic melanosis. It commonly occurs if you have very oily skin, or if you have dandruff on the scalp as well as the alar crease due to a yeast called Malassezia furfur. It is also common if you have insulin resistance or diabetes. So, make sure you check your insulin and blood sugar levels. Avoid scrubbing the skin and always apply a sunscreen. Your dermatologist may prescribe tacrolimus or ketoconazole-based creams.

3. What can I do to lighten my dark inner thighs?

Some of the causes of dark inner thighs are fungal and yeast infections, post-inflammatory hyperpigmentation as a result of skin disorders or infections, friction due to tight clothes, rubbing of thighs in case of those who are overweight, allergy to elastic of inner wear and acanthosis nigricans. One has to identify the cause and treat it. Treating any fungal or yeast infections, if you have them, is necessary. Check for diabetes, insulin resistance and PCOS and make sure to reduce weight if you have to and maintain your BMI below 25. Opt for loose cotton clothes and go for cotton panties with cloth rolled over elastic instead of tight elastic ones. Do not use corticosteroids, retinol or hydroquinone in this region. Your dermatologist may prescribe skin-lightening creams or also do chemical peels and Laser treatments if necessary.

4. I have recently developed dark bluish-black patches all over my cheeks and neck. I have applied various creams, but nothing seems to work. Is this segmentation and how can it be treated?

Hyperpigmentary disorders called lichen planus pigmentosus, Riehl's melanosis, pigment contact dermatitis and ashy dermatoses can result in bluish-black patches over the skin on the exposed parts of the body. You will need to consult a dermatologist for a proper diagnosis and treatment plan. Repeated and frequent sun exposure, allergy to cosmetics, hair dyes, perfumes or any fragrance-based products, some medicines especially those containing heavy metals and bhasmas, certain foundations and concealers, renal or liver disorders and hypothyroidism are some of the common causes. One has to identify the cause, treat it and eliminate the aggravating factors. A few sessions of Q-switched Nd:YAG Laser or Pico Laser will get rid of the pigmentation but this may take six to eighteen months.

5. What are the various causes of hyperpigmentation on the face?

Apart from the reasons mentioned above, the other common causes for increased pigmentation on the face are post-inflammatory hyperpigmentation due to trauma, friction or a skin disorder, hormonal imbalances caused by pregnancy, menopause, hypothyroidism, hyperthyroidism, insulin resistance, Addison's disease, etc., stress and smoking leading to free radical accumulation, vitamin B3 or niacin deficiency or vitamin B12 deficiency and chronic renal failure or liver disorders.

6. What can one do for facial pigmentation?

Any kind of hyperpigmentation is bound to increase with sun exposure. UV rays and infrared rays of the sun can stimulate the melanocytes (pigment-forming cells) to produce more melanin, thereby causing increased pigmentation. Hence it is mandatory to strictly avoid sun exposure if one has hyperpigmentation anywhere on the skin. It is best to wear protective clothing, dark glasses, and wide-brimmed hats when out in the sun. Make sure you apply a sunscreen (with both UVA and UVB protection) with a minimum of SPF 30, PA++++ every day. Have a lot of vitamin C in your food. Include lime, lemon, oranges and berries in your routine diet.

Consult your dermatologist before buying any skin-lightening cream off the shelf. Some of them may contain steroids, which can be unsafe for your skin in the long run. Others may have hydroquinone, a skin bleaching agent that may again cause more pigmentation if used for a long time. Creams containing vitamin C, niacinamide, kojic acid, arbutin, liquorice, glycolic acid and flavonoids are safe. Your dermatologist will identify the cause and treat it accordingly. Chemical peels and treatment with Q-switched Nd:YAG Laser are done for pigmentation that doesn't lighten with creams.

7. Are there any important don'ts if one has hyperpigmentation?

You should avoid scrubbing or using any kind of loofahs as they result in friction leading to hyperpigmentation, any kind of scented or fragrant products, hair dyes, unknown ayurvedic bhasmas, sugar, steam or sauna, swimming during the day in an outdoor pool, sun, smoking and stress.

8. I have dark brown patches on my cheeks. I have used various creams but nothing seems to work. Is it melasma or pigmentation? Should I opt for Laser treatment?

Melasma is a form of hyperpigmentation. It occurs due to hormonal imbalance, oral contraceptives, progesterone or excessive sun exposure or it may be genetic. It is also common during pregnancy when it is called chloasma. It is seen as a butterfly pigment on the cheek and the nose. It could be light to dark brown in colour. It could spread to the forehead, upper lip, chin, in fact the entire face. If the pigment is deposited in the epidermis, it can be lightened with creams and peels, and it may go completely. However, in most cases, it is dermal (spread to deeper layers of skin) or dermo epidermal. In such cases, it can only be lightened. Serums and creams that reduce the pigment melanin should be used as per your dermatologist's prescription. Glycolic acid peels and retinol peels may also help lighten melasma. Q-switched Nd:YAG Laser done at very low energy sometimes helps lighten melasma. However, melasma is known to recur. One beach holiday without adequate sun protection and the pigmentation can come back with a bang. Hence it is extremely important to use a sunscreen every single day, whether indoors or outdoors and whether it is sunny, cloudy, rainy or snowing. It is mandatory to reapply the sunscreen every two hours. Opt for a broad-spectrum tinted sunscreen for adequate

protection from UVA, UVB, visible light including blue
light and infrared rays.

**9. I used to wear spectacles but recently had Lasik surgery.
Constantly wearing glasses has left marks on the bridge
of my nose and under my eyes. It looks terrible. How can
I get rid of these marks?**

Constant friction due to your spectacles has resulted in
localized pigmentation of your skin. Apply a sunscreen
in the day, keep the skin hydrated with a moisturizer
and avoid rubbing or scrubbing the area. At bedtime,
use a cream containing vitamin C along with any of
the botanical skin-lightening agents such as kojic acid,
arbutin, liquorice or pycnogenol. You could go for
a spot tretinoin peel or treatment with Q-switched
Nd:YAG Laser.

**10. All my friends are getting Laser toning done. How
long can it be done safely?**

Laser toning is done either with a Q-switched Nd:YAG or
Pico Laser to effectively correct sunspots, acne scars, post-
inflammatory hyperpigmentation, uneven skin tone and
patchy skin. The Laser energy breaks down the accumulated
pigment, giving a lightening effect. It also bleaches facial
hair. It can be done once in six weeks. You must make sure
you hydrate the skin by using a moisturizer and always use
sunscreen when you are doing Laser toning. We usually do
six to eight sessions at six-weekly intervals and then give it
a break for a couple of months.

CHEMICAL PEEL

The most common procedure for hyperpigmentation is a chemical peel. Let us understand chemical peels a little more.

1. What is a chemical peel?

A chemical peel is a procedure that involves the application of a solution to the skin in a controlled manner to improve skin tone, blemishes, acne, dilated pores and skin firmness. The solution may be an acid, fruit extract, botanical extract or even milk extract.

2. What are the different types of chemical peels?

Chemical peels are divided into three types based on the depth of the procedure: superficial, medium and deep. We do not do deep peels on Indian skin for fear of scarring and burns. Superficial and medium depth peels can be safely done on Indian skin.

Superficial peel: It removes all or parts of the upper layer of the skin (epidermis). It is a light chemical peel. It is used to improve colour and texture of the skin, and reduce mild photoaging, superficial pigmentation and acne.

Alpha hydroxy acids are most commonly used for superficial peels. Glycolic acid is obtained from sugarcane and is used for anti-aging, blemishes and uneven skin tone. Mandelic acid is obtained from bitter almonds and is used for patients with sensitive or dry skin and with acne or blemishes. Lactic acid is obtained from milk and is used for patients with sensitive skin to improve uneven skin tone and hydrate the skin. Other AHAs that can be used are tartaric acid and citric acid. Beta hydroxy acid or salicylic acid peels are used to unclog pores, reduce whiteheads and blackheads, and to reduce the size of dilated pores. TCA (10 to 25 per cent), Jessner's solution, resorcinol and pyruvic acid (alpha ketoacid) can also be used for superficial chemical peels.

Medium depth peel: It removes the upper layer of skin (epidermis) and the upper part of the middle layer of skin (dermis). TCA (35-40 per cent) is used for medium depth peels. It is used to improve the appearance of the skin, skin texture, and to treat photoaging skin.

3. Can you see results after one peel?

You may see a temporary glow with one peel, but for the desired results, a series of four to eight peels may be required at two- to five-week intervals.

4. What are the side effects of peels?

If you do a chemical peel on very flaky, dry skin or severely tan skin, or if you do not take proper care after the peel procedure, there is a risk of redness, swelling, flaking of skin and increased pigmentation, which can last for up to a week or more. Always get peels done by a professional and be mindful of aftercare.

5. How long does a chemical peel take?

The entire peel procedure takes ten to fifteen minutes. Peels are lunchtime procedures and one can go back to work immediately after treatment with adequate sun protection. So, it is one of the quickest skin treatments available.

6. Does the skin become sensitive after a chemical peel?

Choosing the right peel for your skin along with proper post-peel care will never make your skin sensitive.

7. How long will the skin-peeling after a chemical peel last?

After a medium depth peel, skin will start peeling from the third day for up to five to ten days. Do not remove/peel the skin however tempting it may be. Prematurely peeling the skin will prevent it from healing and lead to post-inflammatory hyperpigmentation.

8. Who should not do a chemical peel?

If you have a history of abnormal scarring, if you are taking any medicines that are photosensitive, if you stay out in the sun all day or if you have a herpes virus infection, you should not do a chemical peel. If you have a known history of allergy to any peeling agents, then you should not do a chemical peel.

9. I am using tretinoin cream. When should I stop using it if I'm to do a chemical peel?

Tretinoin causes dryness and irritation, so you should stop the application of the product three days before and three days after the peel as advised by your dermatologist to avoid excessive exfoliation, peeling or irritation. Its use may be resumed when there is no irritation.

RAPID FIRE

1. Will my pigmentation disappear if I scrub regularly?

On the contrary, frequent or vigorous scrubbing leads to friction-induced pigmentation. So please avoid scrubbing regularly.

2. Once I get treated for pigmentation, it will never come back?

That's not true. Hormones, sun exposure, pollution, etc. may cause recurrence of hyperpigmentation.

3. Are Lasers a permanent solution for hypeprpigmentation?

If you are very careful and avoid all the aggravating factors causing hyperpigmentation, you may not get a relapse most of the times. But it may not be possible to treat every type of hyperpigmentation with Lasers.

4. Can Laser treatment for hyperpigmentation thin the skin?

Not if the right parameters and correct wavelength are used and a qualified professional operates the Laser.

5. Can Lasers cause burns and scars?

Yes, if the wrong Laser parameters are used or if the patient steps out in the sun immediately after Laser or doesn't follow post-Laser care strictly.

18

Skin Aging

'Nature gives you the face you have at twenty. Life shapes the face you have at thirty. But at fifty you get the face you deserve.'

—Coco Chanel

There are stories of Cleopatra having used apple cider vinegar to tone her face and honey as a moisturizer.

The pulp that comes out in the process of making wine was first used in Thracian times as a powerful antioxidant and called the elixir of youth.

In the late nineteenth century, a concert pianist was developing frown lines which led her mother, Margaret Kroesen, to develop a system of clear tape that could be worn at night to help reduce wrinkles.

The first cosmetic cream which claimed to reverse the signs of aging was created by Florence Wall in 1927.

Apparently, it contained glandular secretions from a tortoise.

Retinol was discovered in 1909 and first made in 1947. And today, it is the most sought-after antiaging ingredient in skincare products.

In the early 1800s, Dr Justinus Kerner discovered the botulinum toxin (commonly known by its trade name Botox) while studying a batch of undercooked blood sausages that had killed several people in Germany. Instead of studying it under a microscope, he injected himself with the toxin to better understand the effects. Research continued throughout the 1950s and 1960s, and finally in 1978, Botox was established as a drug for many disorders such as cervical dystonia, cerebral palsy etc. In 1987, Dr Jean Carruthers finally discovered the cosmetic uses of Botox.

In recent times, leech therapies, bird poop, snake venom, snail mucin and even semen facials are all becoming popular anti-aging treatments though a lot of research is still needed when it comes to these therapies.

1. What is the process of skin aging?

Skin aging is the result of extrinsic as well as intrinsic aging. Intrinsic aging occurs naturally as we age and is genetically determined. Oxidative stress, glycation, inflammation and genetic mutations are responsible for intrinsic aging. Extrinsic aging, on the other hand, depends on our lifestyle and the environment. Extrinsic factors such as sunlight, blue light, smoking, alcohol, stress, pollution, irregular sleep, unhealthy diet, too much sugar and lack of exercise can enhance intrinsic aging too. As a part of the physiological process, the cells in the lower part of the epidermis reach the surface within twenty-eight days in children and young adults. This cell renewal cycle slows down to forty to sixty days for people above the age of forty. What actually happens is that as we age, dead skin cells shed more slowly and there is a build-up of old cells on the skin surface. The turnover of new skin cells decreases. This leads to dull, flaky skin. The moisture content in the skin reduces due to disruption in the protective lipid layer of the skin and a reduction in hyaluronic acid content in the skin. Therefore, the skin becomes dry and dehydrated. The production of new collagen fibres slows down and older fibres shrivel up. The elastin fibres lose their spring too. This results in skin sagging, thinning and cracking, and the appearance of fine lines and wrinkles.

Telomeres are present at the ends of DNA strands, like plastic caps at the end of shoelaces, and protect the DNA. As the telomeres shorten, DNA gets damaged and can no longer do its job well, leading to early aging. Telomeres shorten as we age, but can also be shortened by stress, unhealthy diet, lack of exercise, smoking, obesity and pollution.

2. How can one prevent facial aging?

It is not possible to prevent facial aging because aging is a natural process of the body. But we can prevent early signs of aging by following a healthy lifestyle, which includes a healthy sugar-free diet, exercise, stress management, and adequate and timely sleep. A proper skincare routine, including using sunscreen 365 days of the year, irrespective of snow or rain, is mandatory even if you have good genes. Keep away from pollution as much as possible. Avoid alcohol, aerated drinks, smoking, Juul and vaping. Get timely preventative skincare treatments done by a qualified dermatologist.

3. Is it important to use a night cream after the age of thirty?

It is important to use a sunscreen in the day and at least a moisturizer at bedtime. Your moisturizer may contain active ingredients or your night cream could contain moisturizing ingredients. On days that you are very tired and skip applying a night cream, do not forget to at least remove your make-up.

4. Does retinol help reverse fine lines if one is in one's twenties?

Retinol is a vitamin A derivative that helps in collagen remodelling and firming the skin. However, deep, formed lines and wrinkles may not disappear with a retinol cream or with any cream for that matter. You may opt for tiny doses of botulinum toxin, microneedling with platelet-rich plasma (PRP) therapy or fractional Laser treatment to get rid of fine lines. Retinol is a great ingredient to prevent fine lines and can be safely used from the age of eighteen. It is, however, unsafe to use during pregnancy.

5. Do topical anti-aging creams actually work? Or are they just hype and marketing?

Yes, they certainly do, provided you begin using them before the damage is done. One should start using an anti-aging, anti-wrinkle cream before the wrinkles appear. The best age to start is thirty years. Once you develop deep wrinkles, do not expect a miracle cream to erase the wrinkles. That miracle can only happen with rejuvenation and resurfacing Lasers such as ResurFX or with botulinum toxin and fillers.

6. Do night creams work better or day creams, or should one use a mix of both?

Our skin does not know the difference between day and night. It works 24x7 to repair itself. So it doesn't matter whether you choose a night cream over a day cream or vice versa. Yes, day creams often have SPF, so they have that added benefit when used in the day. Some night creams, on the other hand, have an ingredient such as retinol, which should not be applied during the day since the efficacy reduces with exposure to light. For any cream to work well, the minimum amount of time it should be on the skin is four hours. So, applying an anti-aging cream at night has the benefit of staying on the skin for a longer time and getting absorbed slowly while day creams have their own role of protecting you from sunlight, dust and pollution, as well as hydrating your skin.

7. What are the active ingredients one should look for in creams? Does it matter if one goes for a serum, gel or cream?

You should look for retinol, hyaluronic acid, peptides, coenzyme Q10, resveratrol, Argireline, green tea, coffee berry, curcumin, vitamin C, vitamin E, glycolic acid, etc. in anti-aging creams. If you have hyperpigmentation, then look for skin-lightening ingredients such as liquorice, kojic acid or coffee berry in addition to other anti-aging ingredients.

Apart from creams, one can apply serums and gels on the skin. However, the question is which one would best suit our skin type. Serums are water-based liquids that contain active anti-aging and skin-lightening ingredients such as peptides, antioxidants, vitamin C, etc. in higher concentrations. They are not heavy and do not contain occlusive moisturizing ingredients such as petrolatum or mineral oil that prevent water from evaporating.

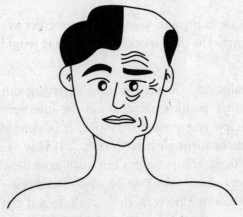

Young face versus aged face

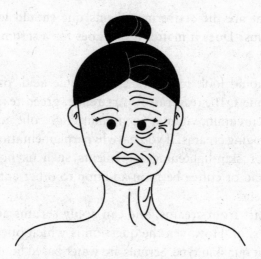

Serums penetrate the skin faster. They are good for all skin types but for those with normal or dry skin, a moisturizing cream is a must in addition to a serum. Creams are great for moisturizing the skin. They are better than serums for people who have very dry skin, while gels are good for those with oily skin.

8. There are many anti-aging home remedies available on the internet. Do they work? If yes, what would be your pick?

I personally do not like the idea of trying out a home remedy after reading about it on the internet. It is not like a recipe you want to try out, it is your skin. You cannot experiment with your skin. It is best to consult a dermatologist before trying out such remedies. But yes, if your grandma asks you to apply turmeric, yoghurt, honey, besan or aloe vera, these are safe and can be tried.

9. Are expensive creams better than inexpensive ones, and what is the right way to apply an anti-aging cream?

One need not spend on a very expensive anti-aging cream. The ingredients must be right, and the cream should suit your skin type as well as the climate. Retinol and glycolic acid-based creams should be applied at night. A pea-sized amount is enough to cover the entire face. Other night creams that have more moisturizing ingredients can be liberally applied. Dab the cream on the entire face and rub it into the skin using gentle circular strokes.

10. Do men and women age differently? Most marketing is targeted towards women rather than men. Why is that?

Men have thicker skin, more sweat and sebaceous glands, and an increased collagen density. So, men generally age more slowly than females. Also, females have reduced oestrogen closer to menopause and after menopause. This dries their skin more and increases the process of skin aging. Women typically start using sunblock and moisturizers at an early age, which delays the process of skin aging. Men, on the other hand, tend to be more careless, and do not use creams and sunscreens regularly. So, in men who do not lead a healthy lifestyle or use sunscreens at an early age, wrinkles and lines may appear sooner.

11. What is your go-to advice for fighting signs of aging?

The first and most important piece of advice is to use a sunscreen regularly even on a cloudy or rainy day, and you must use at least half a teaspoonful for the face and neck. If you are out in the sun for more than two hours, you need to reapply the sunscreen. The second thing is to use a moisturizer because if you do not hydrate your skin well, it tends to develop lines and wrinkles faster, and the skin also becomes more sensitive. Do not forget to use a sunscreen and moisturizer on your neck, arms, hands and feet. An under-eye cream is a must to hydrate the thin skin under the eye. Lead a healthy lifestyle, eat healthy food, sleep on time, avoid sugar, alcohol, and smoking, include at least half an hour of exercise in your daily routine and, finally, learn to deal with stress without letting it get the better of you. We need to practise a holistic approach towards youthful skin.

12. I always thought consuming sugar leads to diabetes. But I read in your book *Skin Rules* that sugar can cause aging too. How is that?

Sugar triggers a process called glycation. Here, sugar molecules bind to collagen and elastin fibres and form advanced glycation end-products. This destroys the collagen and elastin fibres, resulting in premature wrinkles, fine lines and uneven skin tone.

13. Will smoking three cigarettes a week impact my skin?

Smoking just one cigarette a month will also impact your skin negatively. Nicotine is known to increase the free radicals and matrix metalloproteinases in the skin, leading to breakdown of collagen and elastin fibres. It also causes increased melanin synthesis and reduces circulation. Thus, the skin becomes pale, patchy and dull, fine lines and wrinkles appear, pores become more dilated and the face begins to sag. Hence it is best to give up smoking.

14. What is the right age to start anti-aging treatments?

Simple anti-aging treatments such as chemical peels and microneedling can be done in your twenties. PRP and microneedling can be done in your early thirties; radio frequency skin tightening in your mid-thirties; all of these and fillers, botulinum toxin and HIFU from your late thirties; and all of these and thread lifts in your forties and above. All in all, there is no particular age for doing these treatments; if there is a requirement, you can do the treatment. Do not be obsessive and overdo any treatments. Taking baby steps from your thirties will keep you aging gracefully and youthfully.

15. Will Morpheus 8 treatment result in skin tightening?

Morpheus 8 is a radio frequency micro-needling device. Other devices similar to Morpheus 8 are Secret, Endymed, etc. Fine microneedles enter the skin along with radio frequency energy to stimulate collagen, tighten the skin, and reduce pore size and acne scars. Four to eight sessions are done at one-month intervals. The treatment is safe. There is redness and swelling for about twenty-four to forty-eight hours post treatment, and one is advised to strictly avoid sun exposure for about five days post treatment. When combined with PRP, the results are even better.

16. What treatment is good for sagging skin on the face?

The face comprises five layers: bone, deep fat, muscle, superficial fat, and skin. As we age, the bone begins to resorb, the deep layer of fat is lost, muscles become thin and the ligaments that hold the structure get attenuated. Thus, there is little support for the superficial fat layer and the skin. The skin begins to lose its elasticity and the collagen fibres that form the framework of the skin degrade. All these changes together lead to sagging of skin.

When the face skin just begins to sag in your early thirties, radio frequency skin tightening is a good treatment option. In your mid-thirties, you may opt for a combination of radio frequency and high-intensity focused ultrasound (HIFU) treatment. Both these procedures stimulate collagen production and help in skin firming. If the level of sagging is more, one may opt for thread lifts. I usually do thread lifts in people who are above thirty-five. If there is volume loss, filler injections are the best option to restore the foundation and recreate the pillars of support. Again, fillers can be done from any age, but usually people complain of sagging in their late thirties or forties. Fillers can also be done in the fifties, sixties or seventies, but it is always better to start early to prevent the foundation from crumbling.

17. I am thirty-four years old. Can I take baby Botox for crow's feet or is it too early to start Botox?

You can take tiny doses of botulinum toxin around your eyes for the crow's feet to disappear or soften. There is no age restriction for using botulinum toxin. When you see lines and if they bother you, take the injections. However, in my clinic, I usually start botulinum toxin injections for those in their mid-thirties, unless the person has bulky masseter muscles, bruxism or suffers from migraines, which can be treated at a young age too. It does not do any harm. The key is not to overdose. Keep it natural. The effect of botulinum toxin lasts for about four to six months after which you will need to get reinjected. However, if you do not repeat the injection, your lines will not worsen, they will only revert to the state they were in when you started.

18. I am considering Botox injections for my underarms because I sweat a lot. How safe are these injections and will I have any trouble in moving my arm?

It is extremely safe to get botox injected in your underarms if you sweat a lot. Depending on the dose, sweat secretion will reduce or completely stop for six to eight months. However, the injections need to be repeated every six to eight months to prevent the underarms from sweating again.

19. What should I do for forehead lines?

Forehead lines are formed due to hyperactivity of the frontalis muscle. Tiny doses of botulinum toxin will get rid of forehead lines for four to six months. Once the effect wears off, the lines reappear, so you will need to repeat the botulinum toxin injections, if you want. For deep static forehead lines that do not disappear with botulinum toxin, very light fillers may be injected.

20. If I stop using fillers and Botox, will my face sag more?

This is a common misconception. Botulinum toxin and fillers are well-researched, US Food and Drug Administration (FDA)-approved products.

Botulinum toxin is a purified protein derivative of Clostridium tetani. It is injected for the treatment of several medical conditions such as cerebral palsy in patients as young as ten, cervical dystonia, migraines, etc. When injected into specific muscles of the face, it relaxes those muscles and softens wrinkles such as forehead lines, crow's feet, frown lines, bunny lines on the nose, popply chin, smoker's lines around the lips, bulky lower jaw and neck bands. These days it is also given for bulky trapezius muscles and bulky calf muscles. If you stop injecting Botox, the muscles revert to the state they were in at the beginning of the treatment. The lines and wrinkles do not worsen.

Hyaluronic acid fillers are available as pre-filled syringes in doses of 1 ml. They are not the same as botox. They are injected to volumize certain areas of the face such as hollow under eyes, hollow temples, hollow cheeks, depressed forehead, depressed nose, depressed chin, thin lips and wrinkled hands. They are also injected to recreate the jawline or lift a sagging face. Hyaluronic acid is bio-stimulatory. It stimulates fibroblasts in the skin to produce more collagen. Hence lines, wrinkles or sagging on the face will not worsen if you stop the filler injections. Your face will always look better than when you first started injecting the fillers.

21. My dermatologist has suggested that I do fillers as I have lost a lot of weight, and my cheeks are looking hollow. I'm scared of getting them done because I see people with huge apple cheeks and duck lips, which makes them look very plastic and artificial.

It is sad that we do see a lot of pillow faces, duck lips, abnormally filled cheeks, lips, chin and even under eyes. This happens due to over filling the face with a lot of products. Injecting fillers into the face is a work of art and science blended together. You must choose an injector who is well trained and board certified and has an aesthetic eye as well as a skilled hand. Choosing your injector based on the cost of fillers is the worst thing to do. Fillers, when injected in the right quantity and proportion can make one look fresh, youthful and aesthetically pleasing. Go slow, do not over-inject and let your physician sculpt your face, keeping it natural.

22. I am twenty-six years old, and I look tired all the time despite sleeping well. I think I have dark circles, but I have also had sunken eyes since I was in my teens. What can I do to stop looking tired?

Because you have had sunken eyes since you were in your teens, the bones under your eyes, namely, your orbital rim and maxilla, must be genetically concave. This leads to a shadow cast under the eyes, making you look tired. Opt for hyaluronic acid filler injections under the eyes to fill in the hollow. This makes you look fresh and youthful all the time. Too much filler under the eye can make the eyes look small. So, the quantity injected should be just enough to correct the hollows. Anyone above the age of twenty can get these filler injections done.

23. What are the side effects of filler injections?

Hyaluronic acid fillers are very safe and forgiving. In case you don't like the result or if there is a rare complication, it can be dissolved with the help of a medicine called

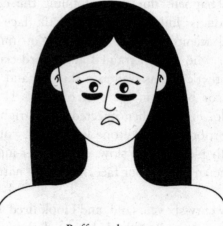

Puffy under eyes

hyaluronidase. Immediately after the filler injection, there may be a bit of swelling, especially when done under the eyes or on the lips. Bruising can occur since the face is full of blood vessels, but a bruise will last for only five to ten days. Both these effects are temporary. You should plan your fillers such that you have no important event or occasion in the following two weeks. Nodules, lumps and bumps are rarely seen and can be dissolved easily if they occur.

24. What is the best treatment for neck lines?

If you have vertical neck bands, botulinum toxin is the best option. The effects last for about four to six months. If you have horizontal lines, low G prime fillers or skin boosters can help. You can also have radio frequency microneedling and HIFU done to tighten the skin.

25. I have a double chin although I have managed to lose quite a bit of weight. Should I opt for surgery or is there a non-surgical option?

If there is a lot of fat in your submental area (double chin), liposuction is the best treatment option. But if it is pinchable fat, you could consider non-surgical options such as cryolipolysis or injection lipolysis, both of which are US FDA-approved.

26. What can one do to get rid of smile lines?

We are all born with smile lines, but they become more prominent as we age. You can do any of the skin tightening treatments such as radio frequency, radio frequency micro-needling, fractional Lasers or HIFU. Fillers are injected into the smile lines in the early stages. If the smile lines turn into deep folds, fillers are injected on the outer side of the face to cause a lifting effect and to reduce the smile lines. Thread lifts may also be done.

27. How does one get rid of bags under the eyes?

Eye bags appear either due to fat prolapse or due to fluid retention. If they occur due to fat prolapse as a natural process of aging, they can be surgically removed. In mild cases of fat prolapse, hyaluronic acid fillers may be injected in tiny doses in the groove beneath the fat bulge. This helps camouflage the bulge. If the bags are due to fluid retention, it is better to avoid salt, sugar, alcohol and smoking. Lymphatic drainage massage may help temporarily.

28. What is a vampire facial?

Vampire facials or PRP facials are a cosmetic procedure that must be done either by a qualified doctor or under medical supervision. The doctor will first draw a vial of blood from your body (like a simple blood collection for blood tests). This blood is centrifuged to differentiate the plasma and platelets from the blood. It is then injected back into your face. These platelets have many nutrients and growth factors that stimulate stem cells and collagen growth.

PRP therapy can be combined with microneedling for better skin regeneration. Microneedling creates channels in the skin that facilitate easy penetration of growth factors, mesenchymal stem cells, cytokines, platelets and other healing components present in the PRP serum into the deeper layers of the skin. This helps boost collagen and elastin fibres and improves the texture and elasticity of skin.

29. What are the benefits of a vampire facial?

Platelet-rich plasma treatment, also known as a vampire facial, helps reduce pore size and fine lines. It is a good preventative anti-aging treatment as it boosts collagen fibres and keeps the skin firm. It also helps reduce acne scars, chicken pox scars, surgical scars, burn scars and stretch marks when combined with radio frequency microneedling or fractional Lasers.

30. Is there any downtime with a vampire facial?

There is a little redness and swelling for twenty-four to forty-eight hours after the procedure. You should protect the skin from sun exposure, apply sunscreen every two hours and avoid using make-up and medicated products for twenty-four hours. It takes at least three months for your skin to show results. At least four to six sessions spaced a month apart are required to obtain the best results.

31. I am forty-two years old. Will I benefit from Exilis or Endymed radio frequency treatment?

Endymed or Exilis are US FDA-approved, non-invasive devices that use radio frequency energy to tighten the skin. Radio frequency energy is sent to multiple layers of the skin simultaneously, which stimulates the synthesis of collagen and elastin. The treatment is painless and requires no downtime. It is a simple, painless, safe, non-surgical lunchtime procedure that feels like a warm massage to the person undergoing it. Usually, treating the face requires thirty minutes while treating both the face and neck requires forty-five minutes for one session. There are no side-effects, and you can walk back to work immediately after the procedure. Depending on the type of device, you may need four to six sessions. You can see results two to three months after the procedure, and the effect lasts for about a year.

32. What is the difference between HIFU and radio frequency treatments? Both are said to be for skin tightening.

While radio frequency treatments use radio frequency energy to heat the deeper layers of the skin, HIFU and Ultherapy use high-intensity focused ultrasound to heat the deeper layers of the skin. Both are intended to stimulate collagen fibres. HIFU also targets the superficial fat layers just below the skin. HIFU is generally recommended for slightly mature skin. A combination of radio frequency and HIFU work wonders in skin tightening. HIFU also has no downtime, but it is slightly painful and requires an anaesthetic cream to be applied on the treatment area for at least forty-five minutes before the procedure in order to alleviate pain.

33. Are thread lifts safe? How long does the effect last and at what age can I start? I am twenty-six and my skin has already started sagging.

Thread lifts are done by inserting medical-grade thread material into your face and then 'pulling' the thread to lift and tighten your face. The various thread materials available are polydioxanone (PDO), poly-L-lactic acid (PLLA) and polycaprolactone (PCL). These are absorbable threads inserted into the skin with fine needles to give a lifting effect. They work by stimulating the body's own collagen to produce newer collagen along the line where they have been inserted. They dissolve in the skin within four to six months. Depending on the type of threads used, they can last for four months to a year. They are usually recommended for people between thirty-five to sixty-five with sagging skin and without excessive fat on their face. There may be pain and swelling as well as bruising for up to a week post the thread lifts. However, this is temporary. This is a lunchtime procedure to lift cheeks, the nose, jawline and even the eyebrows. Threads are also used to treat lax skin under the chin and on the neck as well as the hands. One to three sessions at one-month intervals are needed and the results are seen a month after the treatment. However, as you are only twenty-six years old, you are certainly not a candidate for thread lifts. Try other non-surgical skin tightening options such as microneedling or PRP.

34. What is the difference between CoolSculpting, TESLA Former and Emsculpt?

CoolSculpting uses cryolipolysis energy to freeze stubborn pockets of fat and dissolve them. Double chin, love handles, fat on the thighs and abdomen, and bra fat can be reduced with CoolSculpting in one to three sessions. It is a safe, US FDA-approved, non-surgical procedure and can be done at any age. However, it is not a weight-reduction therapy.

TESLA Former or functional magnetic stimulation (FMS) is procedure that uses electromagnetic energy to tone your abs, building your muscle by burning fat. It is a non-invasive body sculpting, muscle-building treatment for strengthening the abdomen, thighs, calves and biceps and for a buttock lift. It is estimated that a single thirty-minute session of FMS is equal to approximately 50,000 sit-ups or bends. Emsculpt is similar to TESLA Former.

35. What does menopause do to the skin?

In women, oestrogen and androgen output from the ovaries and adrenal glands falls after menopause, resulting in decreased collagen synthesis and repair.

Aging related to the failure of oestrogen production during menopause accentuates intrinsic aging, and together with photoaging may dramatically increase the apparent age of a menopausal woman.

Oestrogen deficiency particularly affects the fibroblasts of the dermis and thinning of the skin is primarily related to a decrease in the production of collagen. The fibroblasts are also responsible for the synthesis of the glycoproteins and hyaluronic acid in the dermis of the skin (which is able to bind water). The decrease in fibroblast activity with age accounts for the decreased dermal hydration.

Skin elasticity decreases with age, but the effect is more marked in women than in men.

RAPID FIRE

1. What are the seven signs of aging skin?

Fine lines and wrinkles, rough skin texture, uneven skin tone, skin dullness, visible pores, blotches and age spots, and skin dryness.

2. Will my wrinkles disappear with snail mucin or snake venom anti-aging creams?

No, formed wrinkles will need botulinum toxin or device-based treatments. Snail mucin and snake venom can be used for preventative anti-aging skincare.

3. Can I do filler injections and fly out the same day?

There is a possibility that your face may swell up more due to high altitudes and cabin pressure in the flights. So, it is always better to wait for twenty-four hours.

4. Can bruises after filler injections or threads be permanent?

No, bruises are temporary. They may last for three days to two weeks. Rarely, a haematoma may take 6 to 8 weeks to resolve. Very rarely, one may develop post-inflammatory hyperpigmentation due to a bruise and will need to be treated

5. I am fifty-six years old, and I want to get rid of lines on my forehead. I read that Botox helps but my dermatologist is asking me to do fillers instead. Why so?

If your dynamic wrinkles on the forehead (lines which appear when you raise your brows) have now become static (lines that persist even when you don't raise your brows), they may not go with Botox injections. Static lines will need a soft filler injection in the creases.

19

Home Use Gadgets

'Skincare has been an ancient tradition which must go on.'

—Dr Jaishree Sharad

Gua sha, meaning to 'scrape away illness', involves using tools such as bian stone, jade or ox horn with lubricant liniment to scrape and rub parts of a patient's skin repeatedly in one direction. The aim is to 'activate blood circulation to dissipate blood stasis', based on TCM theory. Historical records on gua sha go back to the Paleolithic Age, when stones were used to rub parts of the body to help alleviate symptoms of any sickness.

The practice of gua sha in China is about 700 years old, practised since the Ming dynasty (chinaculture.org).

Jade rollers were a part of the beauty ritual among the rich in China since the Qing dynasty in the early seventeenth century.

1. Do jade rollers or gua sha actually do anything?

A jade roller is a stone/crystal rolling device used for facial massage. Gua sha is a handheld gemstone tool used in Chinese medicine to reduce pain or tension in the muscles and joints. Chi or qi when blocked is known to cause muscle aches or stiffness. Gua sha is said to release the chi. Both these tools help drain lymphatic fluid in the skin and reduce puffiness of the face. There are no adequate scientific research/clinical studies to prove their effectiveness. So, one can say that they are basically relaxing tools for the face.

2. Does using a jade roller make the face slimmer?

There are no studies that suggest that using a jade roller reduces fat cells.

3. How often should one use a jade roller or gua sha?

One can safely use jade roller or gua sha every day or every alternate day, for around five minutes.

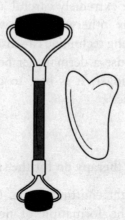

4. Can using a jade roller cause breakouts?

It is very important to clean your jade roller properly after every use. Dirty rollers can trap dirt and oil and clog the pores, leading to breakouts.

5. What is a dermaroller used for?

A dermaroller is a handheld device that comprises a plastic drum-shaped cylinder with tiny needles arranged in rows on it, attached to a handle. Microneedling is done with a dermaroller or dermapen in aesthetic and skin clinics. When you roll it on the skin, it creates tiny channels, which allow specific nanoparticles to penetrate the deep layers of the skin. The needles create tiny wounds, which in the process of healing result in new collagen. It can be used for acne scars, stretch marks, traumatic scars, hair restoration and dilated pores.

6. Can I use a dermaroller at home?

It is not advisable to use a dermaroller at home. First of all, you have to be extremely careful about maintaining aseptic precautions otherwise you will end up with infections. The wrong technique can also lead to scarring. You should not reuse a dermaroller because it is a one-time disposable gadget. It is best to get microneedling done at a skin clinic.

LED MASKS

1. What does light therapy do for the skin?

LED stands for light emitting diode. It increases blood flow, stimulates the formation of new blood vessels, speeds up healing, increases collagen production, and improves the elasticity and texture of the skin. Blue LED light is useful to kill the bacteria that cause acne. It makes the skin look firm and the pores become less visible. Red LED light speeds up healing and stimulates collagen production.

2. Does red light therapy tighten the skin?

Red light LED therapy stimulates healing and collagen production, so it is perfect for anti-aging facials. You see the results after four to five sessions, but they are temporary.

3. What are the side effects of light therapy?

Generally, it is safe for short-term use; the long-term safety is not known. Mild redness can occur. It may also

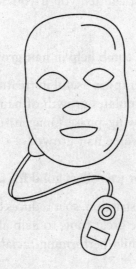

cause damage to the eyes, so it is important to use an eye shield when undergoing LED light therapy.

4. What are the benefits of blue LED light?

Blue LED light is used for the treatment of acne, as blue light reduces the activity of oil-producing glands in the skin and kills acne-causing bacteria.

5. Who should not undergo LED light therapy?

Those on anti-acne medication such as isotretinoin or creams that could be photosensitive, those with skin cancer and those with any eye disorder should not opt for LED light therapy.

6. Can you use LED light device at home?

LED light device for home use is considered safe, but your dermatologist can tell you if you actually need this treatment or not.

7. Does LED light comb help in hair growth?

Yes, LED light therapy is useful in treatment of hair loss. Red LED light stimulates growth of hair follicles. It also promotes the growing phase (anagen) of the hair cycle and thus helps increase hair growth.

8. Are ice facials or ice rollers good for the skin?

Ice causes vasoconstriction, so it reduces blood flow to the skin. Ice rollers are great tools to help alleviate pain and prevent bruises while performing facial procedures like fillers. However, they should be completely disinfected. They also soothe the skin and reduce puffiness. In some patients, they are mood elevators as they calm the skin and make one feel good. Ice rollers do nothing for acne or wrinkles.

RAPID FIRE

1. My face looks puffy in the morning and becomes okay by evening. Is there a quick fix?

Salty meals, alcohol, late nights, hormones and allergies can cause puffiness in the morning. Massage the face with a jade roller or gua sha starting from just below the inner corner of the eye to the ears moving outwards towards hairline and down to the ears. This will assist in draining lymph fluid and reduce puffiness.

2. Can I apply ice on my face every day? Will it prevent acne and wrinkles?

You can use ice every day, but it will neither prevent acne nor wrinkles.

3. Can I use any serum immediately after dermaroller treatment? I have read that it creates openings in the skin and allows easy penetration of serums.

First, avoid using a dermaroller at home. Second, the solutions specially used during dermaroller are microparticles designed to easily penetrate the skin. But, serums have larger molecules, and they may cause irritation or a delayed reaction called granulomas or cysts. So, please wait for twelve hours before using your regular serums.

4. If I use LED light alone, will my acne disappear?

Not at all. LED therapy is only an adjuvant to anti-acne creams and oral medication.

5. Will jade rollers improve loose skin on my neck?

Unfortunately, no. Microneedling radiofrequency is a good option instead.

20

Seasonal Skincare

'Your skin has a mind of its own. It behaves differently in different climates and seasons. And there is no one size fits all.'

—Dr Jaishree Sharad

Our skin behaves differently with every season. The external temperature and humidity play a huge role in dryness or oiliness of the skin. Skin concerns change accordingly. Here are the the common issue in summer, winter and rain.

1. What is the basic skincare routine that one should follow in summer?

Use a sunblock with SPF 30 and reapply every two to three hours if outdoors. Keep yourself hydrated by drinking plenty of water. Eat brightly coloured fruits rich in antioxidants to fight the free radicals in the skin produced due to sun exposure. Make it a habit to wear cotton clothes, wide-rimmed sunglasses and hats and to use umbrellas to prevent sunburn, pigmentation, tanning and allergic rashes. After bathing, dust some antifungal powder (clotrimazole dusting powder is available at any chemist) on your feet, underarms, all body folds and groin. Avoid closed shoes, as wearing them for a long period can lead to fungal infections in the web spaces of the toes. Wear cotton socks if you have to wear closed shoes to work. Change clothes, especially inner wear, at least twice a day. Bacterial and fungal infections of the underarms and groin are more common when one sweats profusely. Avoid wearing damp or sweaty clothes. Make sure your clothes are washed in hot water to kill all germs. Miliaria or prickly heat can often occur especially in covered body parts due to blockage of sweat ducts. Ice, calamine lotion, aloe vera lotion and powder for prickly heat can be applied to soothe skin affected by prickly heat.

2. What are the common skin problems that people face during the monsoons?

Fungal, bacterial and yeast infections, boils and lice are common during the monsoons especially if you wear damp clothes for long hours. Dark and moist environments will breed fungi. It is important to keep yourself dry. If you get wet in the rain, please take a shower and change into dry clothes as soon as you can. Keep a change of clothes and shoes in your office or in your locker in college. Do not tie wet hair as this may lead to yeast infections, dandruff and sometimes even lice. Avoid wearing thick cotton clothes. Wear light georgette or chiffons, which dry easily.

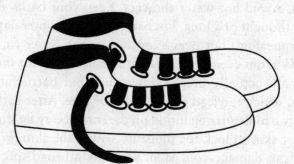

Avoid wearing closed shoes. Wear minimal, preferably waterproof make-up as this will not bleed and clog pores.

3. Can I use the products that I used in summer and during the monsoon in winter?

No, you cannot use products that you use in summer and during the monsoon in winter because in winter your skin needs extra hydration and moisture. Due to low humidity in winter, the lipid structure in the barrier layer of the skin tends to break up. Thus, water is not retained in the skin. Apart from dry skin, other common problems encountered in winter are chapped lips, dandruff, cracked heels, exacerbation of eczema and certain skin disorders such as atopic dermatitis, psoriasis, etc. Thus, it is essential to take care of your

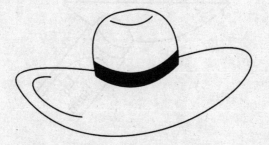

skin. Avoid hot-water showers. Keep your baths short. The thought of a long, hot bath on a cold winter day can be appealing, but over-exposure to hot water can dry the skin out even more. The intense heat of a hot shower or bath actually breaks down the lipid barrier in the skin, which can lead to a loss of moisture. After bathing, apply a moisturizing lotion on the entire body on slightly moist skin to lock the moisture within the skin. Winter sun can damage your skin, so apply a broad-spectrum sunscreen to your face and exposed parts of the skin. Use a lip balm or even ghee for your lips. Do not lick your lips as this will further dry them. At bedtime, use a thick moisturizer that contains fatty acids, cholesterol, and ceramides to repair and moisturize your skin. Hair tends to get frizzy and dry in winter. Don't use hot water to wash your hair and use a good conditioner after every shampoo. Avoid blow drying, ironing and perming as these will cause the hair to become dry and brittle. Wear a scarf or a cap while travelling to protect your hair from sunlight, especially if you have colour-treated hair which can get lighter with sun exposure.

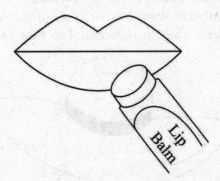

RAPID FIRE

1. My scalp is itchy and dry in winters. What is the reason?

Scalp can get itchy in winters due to poor hygiene, dandruff, low temperatures, exacerbation of inflammatory scalp disorders like seborrheic dermatitis and psoriasis. Please use a 2 per cent ketoconazole or zinc pyrithione-based shampoo twice a week if you have dandruff. Consult a dermatologist.

2. My scalp is very itchy in summers. What should I do?

Accumulation of sweat can breed yeast and fungus. Please use a 2 per cent ketoconazole or zinc pyrithione-based shampoo twice a week. Maintain scalp hygiene. Wash your scalp at least two to three times per week. Make sure you wash your scalp after using hair styling products.

3. What is the remedy for cracked heels in winter that occur despite applying moisturizers?

Use a thick moisturizer which contains ceramides, cocoa butter, and shea butter during the day. Wear cotton socks as far as possible, especially at bedtime. Use a urea and squalene-based moisturizer at night and cover it with socks for better absorption. Use a mild scrub to remove dead cells once a week.

4. My skin peels in winter and even if I apply a moisturizer, it burns.

Use non-foamy, soap-free cleansers. Avoid washing your face more than once or twice a day. Apply a skin repair cream which contains glycerine and ceramides thrice a day. Use a mineral sunscreen. Avoid using all active serums till your skin heals. Take supplements of vitamin E and Omega-3 fatty acids. Avoid exfoliation.

5. Can I use multani mitti or a charcoal or clay face pack in winter to avoid acne?

Clay masks, including multani mitti and charcoal masks, can soak oil and dry the skin further. Best to avoid in winter.

21

Common Skin Conditions

'Your skin is an organ—you would never harm your
heart or lungs in order to approve them. The same
goes for skin.'

—Dr Dennis Gross

Skin is the protective sheath which covers our internal
organs and gives our body a form and shape. It is constantly
subjected to a lot of insult from the environment, climate,
microorganisms, poor lifestyle and internally due to
hormones and illnesses.

Here, I have answered some of the most common
queries on skin issues like fungal infection, eczema, etc.

1. I have some bumps on my cheeks that are not exactly pimples. My cheeks are usually red, and the redness increases when I go out in the sun. Sometimes my nose gets red too. Please advise.

You seem to be suffering from a condition called rosacea. The cause of rosacea is unknown. The symptoms are red areas on the face, a tendency to flush or blush easily, visible small blood vessels on the nose and cheeks, and small red bumps or pustules on the nose, cheeks, forehead and chin (not the same as whiteheads and blackheads). The triggering factors could be spicy food, alcohol, chocolates, temperature extremes, sunlight, stress, anger, strenuous exercise, hot baths, saunas, smoking, etc. Use a mild cleanser to wash your face and apply a broad-spectrum sunscreen daily. Your dermatologist will give you medication in the form of oxymetazoline, metronidazole, tacrolimus, etc.

2. I keep getting ringworm on my inner thighs. It is very itchy. It goes with antifungal cream but comes back when I stop using it.

You need to stop using the antifungal cream as it may contain a steroid. Steroid-based cocktail creams are easily available over the counter and can lead to extremely resistant fungal infections. You must consult a dermatologist and take a proper oral antifungal course of medication, which can last from three weeks to three months and in resistant cases even longer. Do not self-medicate.

Fungal infections are most common in the body folds such as underarms, groin and under the breasts, but may occur on any part of the body. Fungi require a damp and dark environment to grow. When sweat accumulates in the body folds or in the web spaces of your toes when you wear closed shoes or if you wear a helmet or cap all the time and your scalp is sweaty, it forms a good breeding ground for fungi and yeasts. Tinea corporis, tinea pedis (athlete's foot) and tinea capitis are various ringworm infections that can become very resistant if not treated on time.

It is very important to keep your skin dry. After a workout or any activity that involves sweating, you must take a shower and dry yourself completely. Dust an antifungal powder in all the body folds, on your neck and in the web spaces of the toes. Make sure you do not wear sweaty clothes. Opt for loose cotton clothes especially when you are outdoors. If you get wet in the rain, you must change into dry clothes as soon as possible. Avoid staying in damp clothes for long hours.

3. I have multiple small, circular patches on my back and arms. Some of them are white and some are dark. They have been there for two months. There is no itching or pain, but it looks very ugly. Please tell me what to do.

You seem to be suffering from a fungal infection called pityriasis versicolor. Apply an antifungal cream containing ketoconazole twice a day. You can even apply 2 per cent selenium sulphide shampoo on the patches and rinse after fifteen minutes. Use an antifungal powder after your bath. You should keep yourself dry. If you perspire a lot, make sure you change clothes twice a day. Ensure your clothes are washed properly and sun-dried. If the condition persists, you may need an antifungal tablet as suggested by a dermatologist.

4. My skin is very dry, and I often get eczema on my legs and elbows. I also suffer from asthma. What skincare routine should I follow?

You may be suffering from atopic dermatitis since you also have asthma. Eczema can also occur as a result of allergies to fragrance, leather, metal, rubber, dust, pollen, etc. First of all, avoid taking hot-water showers. Keep your baths short. Avoid tub and bubble baths. Use soap-free, fragrance-free body washes. Do not use loofahs and pumice stones. Apply thick, ceramide-based moisturizers at least twice a day on slightly damp skin to lock the moisture within. Avoid alcohol- and paraben-based products. Your dermatologist may prescribe a corticosteroid-based cream, tacrolimus or pimecrolimus for the eczema. Oral medicines may be given in severe cases. Avoid all the triggers and try having a gluten-free, sugar-free diet.

5. I have small, round, hard boils on my face, neck and chest. They do not contain pus, nor are they painful. Some are white and some are flesh-coloured. I showed them to the doctor who said I have molluscum contagiosum. I don't know what that means. Is it a skin disease? What can I do to get rid of it?

Molluscum contagiosum is a viral infection of the skin. It is transmitted by direct contact, either person to person or through shared items such as clothing, towels and washcloths. Furthermore, if a person touches the rash and then another part of his or her body, it can cause spread to that area (known as autoinoculation). If the face is involved, shaving, waxing or threading may cause it to spread. The time from infection to the appearance of lesions can range from two weeks to six months. Usually, there is no itching or any other symptom. However, it is important to get the lesions removed to reduce the rate of spread to other people as well as from one part of the body to another. Removal can be either by simple scraping of the lesions called curettage or removal using radio cautery or cryotherapy, a procedure performed with liquid nitrogen. You must visit a dermatologist for the same.

6. I have developed slightly white patches on my face due to calcium deficiency. I have increased my calcium intake considerably since then, but the patches are still quite prominent. Is there a way to get rid of them?

One doesn't develop white patches due to calcium deficiency. The white patches could be due to an allergy to ultraviolet rays or maybe a condition known as pityriasis alba. There is no specific known cause for this condition, but it is common in those who have sensitive skin (atopic). It is aggravated by sun exposure and lack of vitamin A. You can apply a cream containing 1 per cent hydrocortisone on the white patches at bedtime. You must wear a sunscreen with an SPF of 30 during the day and reapply the sunscreen every three hours. Eat a lot of green vegetables and food rich in vitamin A, i.e., carrots, spinach, yogurt, margarine, eggs, etc. A fungal infection called pityriasis versicolor could also result in light coloured, circular spots on the face, back, shoulders and arms. This too doesn't itch. It's best to consult a dermatologist.

7. I have dark spots all over my hands and legs due to mosquito bites. How can I treat them and how can I prevent the occurrence of new ones?

You seem to be suffering from a condition called prurigo mitis, which is an allergy to mosquito or any insect bites. You will have to wear clothing that covers you fully, especially after 4 p.m. or even during the day if you are in the garden or outdoors where there are a lot of trees and plants. Wearing full sleeves, full pants and socks is the key. At bedtime, use a mosquito net if possible. Mosquito repellent may work to a certain extent, but ensure you are not allergic to it since your skin is sensitive. Do a test patch with mosquito repellent cream first. You may have to apply a corticosteroid cream for the acute allergy to subside. Your dermatologist will prescribe pigment-lightening creams to lighten the marks.

8. I recently went to the Maldives and my skin got burnt. It is dark and is peeling. What can I do?

Sunburn can be extremely painful and uncomfortable even at the mildest stage. Skin damage from a sunburn may be minimal and show up as a mild redness that rapidly resolves, or it can be so severe as to cause blisters with fluid accumulation and peeling of large areas of skin. If you are already sunburnt, apply ice, cold calamine lotion and pure aloe vera gel and keep yourself hydrated. A mild cortisone cream does help in case of severe sunburn. Antioxidants such as vitamins C and E are helpful in curing sunburn. Wear wide-brimmed hats or carry an umbrella for additional sun protection. Minimize sun exposure between 10 a.m. and 4 p.m. when the sun's rays are the strongest. Sunglasses with UV-blocking filters are very important. Wear cotton clothes and preferably full sleeves so your arms are protected from the sun. Increased water intake and protective clothing will help prevent sunburns.

9. I have severe vaginal itching with occasional white discharge. I have taken plenty of anti-itch medicines and applied creams. Nothing helps. What can I do?

Please consult a gynaecologist to rule out infections, allergies or vulvovaginal disorders. A curdy white discharge usually indicates a yeast infection such as candidiasis. A thin white, yellow or greenish vaginal discharge that has a bad odour could imply trichomonas vaginalis. Or you could be suffering from a bacterial infection. Humidity, sweat, improperly washed inner wear and faecal contamination can lead to infections. Some infections are sexually transmitted too. Allergies to soaps and creams, fabric, lubricants and spermicides, sanitary pads, and shaving and depilatory products can cause itching. Hormonal imbalance, menopause and stress can also lead to severe itching. Sometimes there could be atrophy of the vaginal and vulval wall, either due to the physiological process of aging or due to an illness leading to dryness and itching.

Always use fragrance-free, non-irritant, hypoallergenic, soap-free, pH friendly mild cleansers or intimate washes. Wash or wipe the genitals from front to back and use lukewarm water to wash. This is important because cleaning in the opposite direction can make way for bacteria from the anus to the vagina and urethral opening, leading to infection. Make sure you wash your hands with warm water and soap after changing your pad/tampon/menstrual cup. Wear comfortable, clean, loose inner wear. Your inner wear should be washed with hot water and a fragrance-free detergent. The detergent should be thoroughly rinsed out to prevent allergic reactions. Use fragrance-free, glycerine, dimethicone, coconut oil, hyaluronic acid or squalene-based vaginal moisturizers.

10. I pierced my nose a month ago and have been wearing a gold stud in it. There is a painful red bump that has developed in that area. It bleeds on touching and has also developed pus. What should I apply on the infected area?

You seem to have developed pyogenic granuloma. Sometimes when there is trauma to the skin/ cartilage, there is rapid proliferation of capillaries, which results in a reddish bump. Apply mupirocin ointment twice a day. You will also need a course of antibiotics and anti-inflammatory medicines. Hence it would be better to consult a dermatologist. Remove the nose stud for a few days else it will delay the healing. If it doesn't heal, it may need to be cauterized.

11. I have scaly patches on my elbows and knees. They itch at times. Lately, I have been getting a few patches on my legs too, so I am worried. What should I do?

You seem to be suffering from psoriasis, which is an inflammatory disorder of the skin. The cause is not known, but the body's immune system is triggered, which speeds up the growth cycle of skin cells. A normal skin cell matures and falls off the body's surface in twenty-eight to thirty days. But a psoriatic skin cell takes only three to four days to mature and move to the surface. Instead of falling off (shedding), the cells pile up and form lesions. Emotional stress, injury to the skin, some types of infection, reactions to certain drugs or cold dry weather can all be triggering factors. You should use a mild soap or liquid cleanser for bathing. Apply a moisturizer after your bath on moist skin. Also make sure you apply a moisturizer on the scaly patches two to three times a day. Take supplements of evening primrose oil daily. Keep stress at bay by yoga or meditation. If the patches persist, you should consult a dermatologist.

12. I have a tiny white eruption on my face. It is not a whitehead since it doesn't come out if I squeeze it. Sometimes, if I poke it too hard, something pearly white and hard comes out. I have tried various creams, but they don't work. What is the remedy?

You seem to be suffering from milia. These are tiny cysts in the upper layer of the skin. They are formed from a hair follicle (pilosebaceous unit) or sweat gland (eccrine gland) when the skin does not slough off normally but instead remains trapped in a pocket on the surface of the skin. There are no creams or tablets to get rid of them. They need to be extracted with a curette. Get this done by a dermatologist. Do not try to break them on your own as you may develop an infection or be left with dark marks.

BODY ODOUR

1. I never had body odour in the past. But now my sweat smells very bad. Does it have to do with my hormones as I am forty-nine and perimenopausal?

Hormonal changes that occur as part of your natural physiological aging during the perimenopausal age can result in excessive sweating and night sweats. This may lead to body odour. You may consult with a gynaecologist for vitamins or oestrogen-mimicking supplements, etc. Apply deodorants or powder in the armpits. You could also opt for botulinum toxin injections in the underarm skin. This is a safe procedure that can reduce sweating for at least six months and prevent body odour.

2. How can I get rid of body odour?

Body odour occurs when sweat comes in contact with even normal bacteria on your skin. Those who sweat

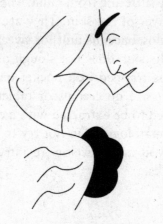

Body odour

profusely are more predisposed to body odour. Body odour can worsen with hormonal changes, heat, sweat, stress, exercise, certain medicines, certain foods like garlic, onions, cabbage, cauliflower, broccoli, MSG and alcohol, or medical conditions such as diabetes, kidney disease or liver disease.

Always keep your skin clean and dry. Take a shower immediately after you exercise. Hair is a breeding ground for bacteria. So, it is better to shave the hair in the armpits and pubic region. Wear clean, dry clothes. Loose-fitting, cotton clothing is better than synthetic fabric. Use deodorants and antiperspirants as and when required. Avoid foods that are likely to increase body odour. Get treated for hormonal conditions or bacterial and fungal infections if any. Find ways to reduce your stress levels. Stress can increase the apocrine sweat secretion. Botulinum toxin, microwave device and radio frequency micro-needling are treatment options that help reduce sweat and body odour.

RAPID FIRE

1. What to do for hives on my body?

Find the culprit and avoid it. Get an allergy test. Consult a dermatologist or an allergy specialist.

2. My toes are itchy, and the web spaces often get white and soggy. What could be the reason?

Yeast or fungal infection of the toes and web spaces. Please keep your feet dry and clean. Avoid wearing closed shoes. Sweat is food for fungus. Consult a dermatologist.

3. The skin on my nose where my spectacles sit has become dark. What should I do?

Change your spectacles. Wear frames that do not have nose pads. Friction or allergy to metal or plastic can cause hyperpigmentation. Your dermatologist may prescribe pigment-lightening creams or chemical peels to lighten the colour.

4. I have syringomas under my eyes. Is there a cream to get rid of them?

Syringomas are tiny, skin-coloured, harmless tumours which occur because of overgrowth of the sweat glands. Laser ablation or cauterization using radiofrequency are the only ways you can get rid of syringomas. However, recurrence is common.

5. I get a lot of itching under my breasts. Is it due to sweat because I am obese and sweat a lot?

Yes, you may be suffering from a yeast infection like candida or a fungal infection. Please keep the area dry. Dust some clotrimazole powder after a shower. Consult a dermatologist for oral antifungal medication as well.

6. Why do I get herpes infection on my lips frequently even if I don't have any physical contact?

Herpes labialis shows up as tiny painful blisters in a particular spot on the lips. The first time it occurs, it could be due to kissing, using an infected towel or even threading. However, subsequent episodes of herpes labialis are not due to contact or kissing. The virus that infected you the first time never dies. It lies dormant most of the time and returns to the same area of the lips which it attacked the first time. It could also recur when one is physically or mentally stressed or has fever. Please consult a dermatologist to avail a proper course of anti-viral medicines.

22

Common Skin FAQs

> 'Skin confidence is the best and cheapest form of make-up one can wear for the most elegant and gracious look.'
>
> —Dr Jaishree Sharad

This chapter has a mixed bag of frequently-asked questions—from pregnancy skincare to male skincare to removal of tattoos. Let's go through them together.

1. I am six months pregnant. What skincare ingredients/ formulas should I avoid?

Retinol/retinoic acid or retinyl palmitate and retinoids such as isotretinoin are extremely unsafe to use during pregnancy as they may cause defects in the brain and spinal cord of the baby. Salicylic acid and benzoyl peroxide, commonly used for acne, can be harmful when applied to large areas of the skin. Hydroquinone and arbutin, which are present in many depigmenting creams, chemical sunscreen contents such as oxybenzone and avobenzone, octinoxate and octisalate are also unsafe. Essential oils of sage and rosemary are also unsafe to use as they can cause changes in blood pressure and a tendency to bleed. Higher concentrations of aluminium chloride found in antiperspirants, parabens, sodium lauryl sulphate and diethanolamine (DEA) found in skin and hair products are also considered unsafe.

2. How can I maintain my skin's natural pH in high temperatures?

The skin's natural pH is between 4.7 and 5.75, which is slightly on the acidic side. High temperatures, pollution and scorching sun can affect your skin. Avoid harsh soaps and cleansers. Soaps are alkaline in nature and alter the pH of your skin. This can lead to dryness, flare-ups of acne and eczemas. Don't use hot water and avoid heavy scrubbing and prolonged baths as this tends to deplete the normal acidic mantle of the skin and cause drying. Moisturize your skin using barrier creams as they help protect the acidic mantle of the skin from environmental damage. Avoid using over-the-counter skincare products such as retinoids, and hydroxy acids such as salicylic acid without the advice of your dermatologist. Use sunscreen as it will protect your skin from both sun and pollution. Apply vitamin C serums or creams that help restore the normal pH of your skin. Follow a proper diet including eating plenty of fruit and green vegetables, which contain vitamins and antioxidants and thus help fight environmental damage and protect the skin.

3. Are all home remedies safe?

No doubt most fruit and vegetables contain alpha hydroxy acids, vitamin A and vitamin C. However, their pH and pka values are different when applied on the skin without processing. That can be more harmful than beneficial to the skin.

Some home remedies you should never rub lemon on the face or using lemon juice in face packs. Lemon has a pH of about 2, so it is very acidic and can damage the protective barrier and alter the pH of the skin, which is between 4 and 5. This can also make the skin more sensitive and lead to rashes and hyperpigmentation. Never use toothpaste on pimples. Toothpaste contains ingredients such as hydrogen peroxide, fragrance, alcohol, baking soda and sorbitol, which dry the skin and result in skin irritation and even chemical burns. Baking soda by itself should also be avoided. Baking soda is extremely alkaline. Not only does it dry the skin, it can also cause certain types of bacteria to grow, leading to

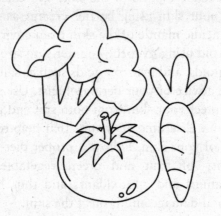

skin infections. Avoid rubbing tomatoes on the skin or using them in masks as they can irritate the skin. Even though their pH is acidic, it does not match with that of the skin. Avoid applying cinnamon or garlic paste on your skin to reduce dark spots or acne. This can actually damage the deeper layers of the skin and cause burns and permanent scarring. If your skin is dry or flaky, or if you are on acne medication, do not use fruit extracts, potato, tomato or lime juice on the skin. These will dehydrate the skin and make it more sensitive. It could even lead to irritation. If you have oily skin, avoid milk cream (malai), milk and oils on the face. These will clog the pores and give rise to more whiteheads. If any of your ingredients are old, or the containers are not clean or your spoons/hands are dirty, you may develop boils or infections.

4. I am a thirty-four-year-old male who leads a healthy lifestyle. I neither smoke nor drink. I eat healthy and exercise. Recently, I have noticed a dark band-like pigmentation on my forehead and the skin feels like it is sagging. What skincare should I follow to at least look my age?

Men too have skin, and they should start skincare right from their teens. You must moisturize your skin and apply a sunscreen every single day. Use a pigment-lightening cream at bedtime. Use a retinol-based serum two or three times a week. You can opt for chemical peels for the hyperpigmentation on your forehead. You may also get radio frequency or high-intensity focused ultrasound (HIFU) skin-tightening treatments since the skin is just about beginning to sag. Fillers, botulinum toxin and thread lifts can also done in men if there is visible sagging.

5. Is male skin different from female skin?

Yes, it is. Men generate about four times more sebum (oil) than females. This is because sebaceous gland activity and composition is affected by androgens, and males have higher androgen levels. This explains why men are more prone to acne and enlarged pores. The baseline sweat output rate of men is 30 per cent higher than that of females. Hence, they are more prone to fungal infections. Men have a decreased ceramide composition in the stratum corneum, which is important for the water barrier function of the skin. Hence they are prone to developing dull and dehydrated skin. Men may have a darker skin tone because of increased baseline pigments such as melanin, haemoglobin and carotenes. Men are more sensitive to UV rays. They have a 16 per cent lower minimal erythema dose threshold which means their threshold to withstanding sunlight is 16% less than females. Hence their skin ages faster. Men have 20 per cent higher collagen density (thickness) and facial bone density. This helps maintain elasticity and gives structural support to the skin. So, there is less sagging. A stronger facial musculature results in deeper expression lines in men.

6. I am a nineteen-year-old male. Can I use my sister's skincare products since I don't know what to use for myself?

Products meant for females can certainly be used by males as well provided they are suitable for their skin type. Therefore it would be better if you consulted a dermatologist because your skin type and skin texture may be different from your sister's.

7. How are male skincare products different from female skincare products?

The packaging is different and some of the night creams may be thicker and packed with a lot of ingredients so that men don't have to layer products. But by and large, most creams are just the same.

8. Why do dermatologists blame stress as the cause of any skin condition from acne to pigmentation to eczema?

When a person is stressed, anxious or angry, the hypothalamus in the brain releases corticotropin releasing hormone (CRH). This in turn stimulates the pituitary gland to release more hormones such as ACTH, which in turn stimulates the adrenal gland to secrete glucocorticoids and catecholamines. The brain also secretes substance P, prolactin and neurotransmitters. All of these send signals to the skin cells. As a response to the signal, various skin cells such as keratinocytes, mast cells and fibroblasts secrete more hormones, which result in exaggerated responses in the existing skin condition. Whether it is acne, rosacea, psoriasis or eczema, all of them increase. The skin barrier is compromised, making the skin sensitive and sometimes dry and dehydrated. There is rapid breakdown of collagen and elastin fibres leading to fine lines and early signs of aging. Hair loss,

Y. Chen, J. Lyga. Brain-skin Connection: stress, inflammation and skin aging. Inflammation & Allergy-Drug Targets. 2014; 13 (3): 177–190. do i:10.2174/1871528113666140522104422.

dark circles and hives can also occur due to stress. So, there is a scientific corelation between stress and the skin.*

9. How can stress be avoided?

Stress is a part of life and every human being suffers from it. However, one must learn the art of coping with stress. While some benefit from meditation and pranayama, others release their stress by exercising, swimming, playing sports, dancing, painting, listening to music or pursuing a hobby. It is a question of giving yourself some me-time every single day.

10. Which beauty products should one always keep with one when one is on the go, and why?

You must keep a moisturizer and sunscreen if you're stepping out in the sun. Also, carry a thermal spring water if you sweat a lot, to clean the face and maintain hydration. And a lip balm to prevent chapped lips.

11. What are the beauty mistakes that one must avoid before a big event or a wedding?

Avoid consuming sugar, alcohol and too much salt to avoid bloating. Do not start using any new skincare products or make-up if you haven't used them before. Any skin procedures should be planned and finished a week before the big day. Do not pop pimples on your

---

* Y. Chen, J. Lyga. Brain-skin Connection: Stress, Inflammation and Skin Aging. Inflamm Allergy Drug Targets. 2014; 13 (3): 177–190. doi:10.2174/1871528113666140522104422

own since this can cause blemishes or scarring that could last for a long time. Instead, consult a dermatologist. Drink enough water and sleep well.

12. I am allergic to regular chemical bleach. Can I get my hair bleached with a Laser instead?

Q-switched Nd:YAG or Pico Laser do bleach dark hair and are better options for bleaching hair, especially if you have sensitive skin or are allergic to chemical bleaching powders. You may do a session once every two months. It is an excellent option for the peach fuzz on your face too.

13. What are skin boosters? My doctor has asked me to go for them now that I am thirty-five years old.

Skin boosters are hyaluronic acid injections and are available under the brand names Juvederm Volite, Profhilo and Restylane Vital. They are injected into the surface layer of the skin and stimulate fibroblasts. Fibroblasts in turn produce collagen and firm the skin over time. They also hydrate the skin and make it look resilient. They are not fillers and do not have the volumizing capacity that a filler has. Multiple tiny injections are given in the skin after numbing it for thirty minutes. Injections are spaced at four weeks for three sessions. Post procedure, the face can be a little bumpy and red at the injection sites with an occasional bruise. All these are temporary and will last for a day or two. Treatment can also be done for the back of the hands and decolletage for hydration and reduction of fine lines.

14. What is a carbon peel? Can I do it before my wedding?

Carbon peel, also known as a Hollywood peel, is a no-downtime procedure that helps rejuvenate the appearance of aging and damaged skin. This gentle procedure is safe on most skin types and is a great way to get a quick skin refresher, giving radiant, glowing skin. It evens the skin tone, reduces the appearance of pigmentation, fine lines and acne scars and makes the skin feel and look more youthful.

A layer of carbon is applied on the entire face like a mask. This is left on for twenty minutes. The Spectra XT Laser is then shot on the entire face through the carbon mask. This helps in deep cleansing, killing microorganisms and reducing the pore size immediately. It also helps reduce whiteheads and blackheads. It gives an instant party glow and is a great alternative to a facial. While it is a great treatment option for brides and grooms, it is always advisable to do the treatment at least four to six weeks before your wedding. If well tolerated, you could repeat it a week before your wedding.

15. I have a tattoo on my arm that I want to remove. How safe is a tattoo-removal procedure and is it really effective?

If you have a black or grey tattoo, it can be easily removed with a Q-switched Nd:YAG Laser. One needs six to eight sessions spaced two months apart to get the tattoo removed completely. Picosecond Lasers are newer Lasers that get rid of coloured tattoos in one to four sessions only. Picosecond at 755 nm is used for blue and green tattoo removal; Picosecond Laser at 532 nm is used for rapid removal of yellow, red and orange tattoos;

and Picosecond Laser at 1064 nm is used for tattoos in darker skin types. Usually, there is no scarring, and the treatment is safe and effective.

16. I either workout or play a sport for an hour every day. Is there any particular care I need to take for my skin?

Skincare both before and after any activity that involves sweating is important. Before playing a sport or working out, remove all make-up and wash your face well. It isn't a good idea to wear make-up and exercise. Sweat mixed with make-up will clog pores and give rise to acne/whiteheads. Apply a good moisturizer. As you exercise, you sweat, and the body as well as skin gets dehydrated. So, you need to hydrate your skin in advance. If you are doing hot yoga, you will need to use a thicker moisturizer. If it is an outdoor workout, you must not forget to apply sunscreen on the face, neck and arms. Use a thermal water mist while you do weights or cardio to clean your skin, clear the sweat and refresh the face with rich minerals. After your workout or sport, make sure you take a shower and cleanse well immediately. Change your clothes. Dirty, sweaty clothes will harbour fungus and bacteria. Moisturize your skin well. Apply a sunscreen if you have to step outdoors.

17. There are so many collagen supplements available in the market in the form of capsules and powders. How effective are they? Will they reduce fine lines and wrinkles and improve skin sagging?

Currently, the research on oral collagen supplements is still ongoing. Indeed, there are many supplements available in the market, but there is a lack of evidence-based data. Some specific formulations have shown to improve very fine lines and the texture of the skin as well as hair. However, there is no improvement in skin sagging. In order to rebuild collagen in your skin, you can take food rich in amino acids such as bone broth, chicken, fish, egg whites, beans, berries, tomatoes and greens. In your twenties, you can opt for chemical peels and microneedling. In your early thirties, you can add platelet-rich plasma therapy in addition to peels and micro-needling. In your mid-thirties, you can add radio frequency and skin booster injections, while in your late thirties, you can add HIFU and hyaluronic acid fillers, which are biostimulatory. In your forties and above, you can do all these treatments to boost collagen.

18. You have always said that sugar, maida and milk are not good for the skin. Can you tell us what food is good for skin?

You must eat five portions of brightly coloured fruit and vegetables every day, including orange, red, green, violet, and yellow fruit and vegetables. These are rich in antioxidants and help fight free radicals. Tomatoes, carrots, apricots, cantaloupe, mango, papaya, pumpkin, and sweet potatoes are rich in lycopene and vitamin A; berries are rich in antioxidants; and citrus fruit, blackcurrants, blueberries, guava, red peppers, parsley, strawberries and broccoli are rich in vitamin C. Avocados are rich in vitamins C and E and in monounsaturated fat, which (like other fats and oils) helps your body absorb certain vitamins, including A, D, E and K. All green leaves are a powerhouse of vitamins. Yoghurt is a good probiotic. Black tea and green tea are rich in flavonoids, which are antioxidants. Seeds and nuts are rich in omega-3 fatty acids. Chicken, lean meat, egg whites, sprouts, tofu, mushrooms, lentils and pulses are rich in proteins. And all of these are great for the skin, hair and nails.

19. I am a make-up artist and am going to start my own studio. Can you give me some tips?

You must use good brands of make-up. Do not compromise on quality for the sake of cost as you wouldn't want your clients to end up with rashes. Avoid using make-up that has expired or changed colour or texture. Eye make-up over six months old should not be used. Always make sure you use sterile brushes, stylers and combs. Keep your muslin cloths and sponges clean. See that they are washed with hot water and dried well before use. Do not touch skin that has a lot of pimples. Ask the client to consult a dermatologist first. If make-up is mandatory for a person with an active infection, you must use separate tools and make-up for him/her. You may also ask them to get their own make-up kit. Always use a moisturizer/sunscreen even before applying a make-up primer.

20. I have a mark left behind by stitches on my face. How can I get rid of it?

Six to eight sessions of fractional Laser treatments combined with platelet-rich plasma therapy and radio frequency microneedling will help reduce or get rid of dramatic scars, surgical scars as well as acne scars. Consult a dermatologist for the best treatment option for you.

RAPID FIRE

1. I have used salicylic acid serum thrice a week last month, but I just found out I am pregnant. Will it harm my baby, or can I continue with the pregnancy?

Please go ahead with your pregnancy. Only very large volumes and high concentrations of salicylic acid used for prolonged periods may have some adverse effect. Most salicylic formulations contain 2 per cent salicylic acid which is perfectly safe.

2. If I plan to conceive, how many months prior should I stop using retinol?

It is better to avoid topical retinoids one month before and oral retinoids such as isotretinoin-3 months before you plan to conceive.

3. Can I apply coconut oil to massage my newborn baby's face?

Oils can sometimes cause milia or infantile acne. So, check with your doctor or do a test patch first.

4. My six-month-old baby has thick flakes of dandruff on the scalp. Should I oil the scalp and remove the flakes?

No, please leave it. The condition is called cradle cap or seborrheic dermatitis. It is better to consult a paediatric dermatologist.

5. My lip corners are turning dark and dry. What can I do?

Allergy to toothpastes or lipsticks, drooling of saliva during sleep, lip licking and vitamin B deficiency can cause dryness and darkening of lip corners. Eliminate the cause and consult a dermatologist. Avoid fluoride-based toothpastes and lip licking. Use a dimethicone and petroleum jelly-based cream over the lip corners, so that it forms a barrier between the skin and your saliva. Take supplements of B complex and vitamin C.

6. Why do lips get sensitive and peel constantly?

Some of the common causes are lip licking, along with allergy to lipsticks, especially the long-lasting matte ones, lip balms containing fragrance, regular and gel nail polishes, gel- or fluoride-based toothpastes, after-mint and cloves, smoking, chewing tobacco and betel nut. Sometimes it could be a result of an inflammatory disorder. Avoid the cause. Keep your lips hydrated. You may use petroleum jelly until you consult your dermatologist.

Acknowledgements

I thank my parents for making me believe in myself and for teaching me to be perseverant, hardworking, honest and kind. I am sure they are watching me from another realm and I hope I am making them happy.

Heartfelt gratitude to Mr Amitabh Bachchan for being my constant source of inspiration, and for his encouragement and support whenever I need it.

I thank all my dearest friends and ardent supporters who have written words of praise for me in this book and all those who couldn't write yet wish well for me. Love you all.

A huge shout out to my editor Gurveen Chadha for being so patient, supportive and understanding apart from encouraging and pushing me to write this book.

Thank you, Milee Ashwarya, from the bottom of my heart and Penguin Random House India too for giving me this grand opportunity again.

Thank you, Pooja Mertia, for making my stunning book cover for the third time.

344 Acknowledgements

Thank you, Neelam Chudasama, for the illustrations in the book.

Last but not the least, my patients and my Instagram family, without your questions on skin and hair care, this book would not have been legit and even possible—I am truly grateful to all of you.

My constant people, you mean the world to me. I thank you all from the bottom of my heart:

- My husband Dr Sharad Sharma, for being my advisor and my rock for three decades now.
- My sister Anupama, my brother Saikarun and my sister-in-law Dipika for being my shoulders to cry on and my best friends too
- My soul children, Aarav and Giana, for being my happiness
- My soul friends, Anju and Riddhima, for always supporting me and encouraging me wholeheartedly in everything that I do
- My assistant doctors and all my staff for being so cooperative, patient and loving
- Papaji, Shweta, Chetan, Archit, Piyali, my grandparents, uncles, aunts and cousins, thank you!